A Guide to TappyBear

How to Use Tappy for Your Child and Yourself

by Patricia Carrington, Ph.D.

Pace Educational Systems, Inc.   Kendall Park New Jersey

Pace Educational Systems, Inc.
61 Kingsley Road
Kendall Park, NJ 08824

A Guide to TappyBear
Copyright © 2008 by Pace Educational Systems, Inc

Edited by Ginny Grimsley
Cover Design by Helen VanLingen
Interior Book Design by John-Dan Key
Tappy Sketch by Kathy O'Malley

ISBN 978-1-60643-872-5

Other Books by Patricia Carrington

The Book of Meditation
Releasing
The EFT Choices Method
Try It On Everything: Discover the Power of EFT
Multiply the Power of EFT

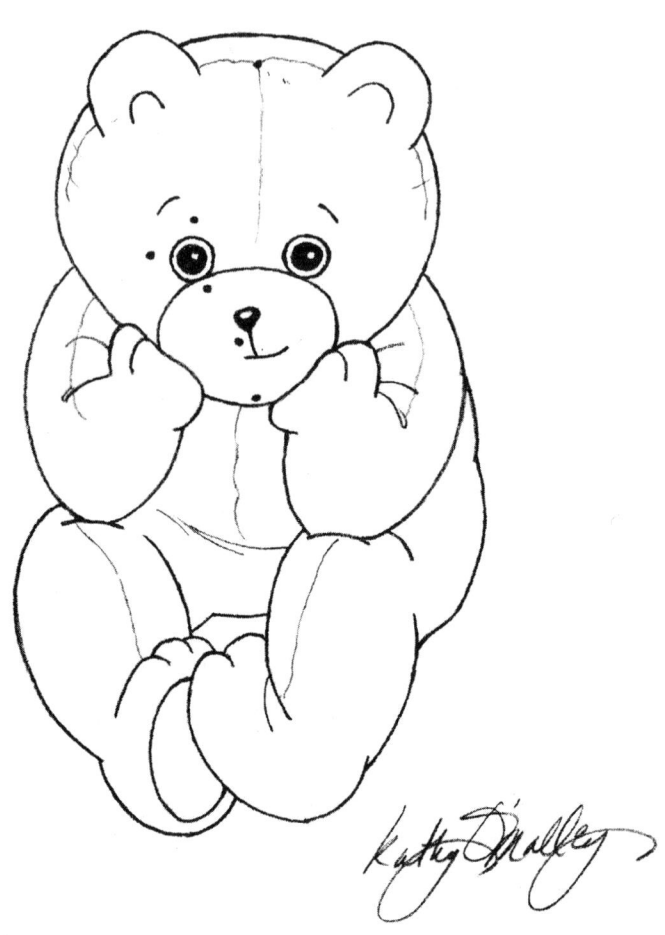

Table of Contents

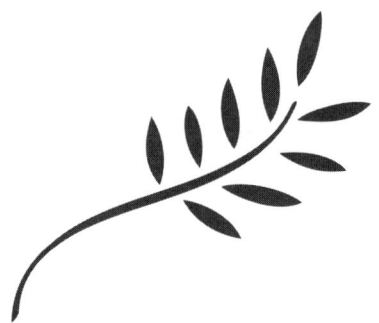

Chapter 1

Meet TappyBear

If you are holding this book in your hands, you may already have met its hero, TappyBear. If so, you may have begun to absorb the warmth, deep compassion and kindly spirit that radiates from his understanding eyes.

Let me tell you more about him.

There are many possible reasons why Tappy's box bore the address that brought him to your doorstep. Tappy might have come here for your nephew who thinks no one likes him, for one of your students whose mother passed away, or for a client who struggles with uncontrolled rage and has not yet been able to respond to therapy. But what you may not yet realize is that the person for whom Tappy is intended could very well be YOU. You may actually be the one whose heart flutters at the thought that he is finally HERE! But whether you ordered TappyBear for yourself or others, know that you have now created the beginning of a wondrous, perhaps even magical, journey.

This book is a guide to help you realize, on a deep level, who TappyBear is — his history, his purpose, and the ways in which he can faithfully serve you and others. But what I'd like you to do at this point is simply *imagine* that TappyBear is here to serve you personally. This is important because nestling up to Tappy and calling him yours for now (or for always) will make all the difference in helping you truly understand what it feels like to have him there at your side when you need a friend. When you have experienced this for yourself, you will come to understand more about how to help others with Tappy.

And so, from here, take Tappy's paw and read on, as though the road you walk is just for the two of you. Here we go…

Life is a journey whose winding path presents us with a variety of surprises. We may be offered a slow river for lazy swimming one moment and find ourselves swatting bats out of our hair the next. Tappy is, for all of us, an open, accepting face and a soft hand to hold as we walk this unpredictable path. His role is to remind us that, no matter where we find ourselves on that journey, *we are not alone*. There is a warm, smiling presence in our lives with whom to share what is beautiful, fascinating, terrifying, or heart-breaking in the world around us. TappyBear is here to remind us to feel the spark of YES! inside us, and to know that the deep ache of our tears is shared. He is here to remind us that when we are truly with *ourselves*, in kindness, we are our *own* loving presence who walks with us always.

Keeping this in mind, hold Tappy up and look him straight in those clear innocent eyes as long as you like. (I'll wait).

Still holding him, whisper to him whatever comes to your mind in warm welcome (again, I'll wait). See how he recognizes you, how his expression says, "Hello, *(say your name here)*! What can we do together? I'm ready to go!"

Now I'd like you to straighten him up as if he's going to the prom. Perk his ears so that they can listen to you fully. Straighten his nose so that it can catch the scent of the path ahead. He's traveled a long way in that confining box to be with you, and (just like the rest of us) he likes to make his best impression when he first meets you and the other new people in his life. So give him a good fluffing up, and watch how he sparkles!

At this point you may be thinking, "This is a bit off target isn't it? This author is presenting this bear as though it were real! What's going on here?"

I understand, but do not worry. My intent here is good, and you will soon understand what it is all about.

Please continue…

What I'd like you to do now is to look deeply into Tappy's eyes and pretend that you see yourself in those eyes — as if his eyes were your own eyes looking back at you with tenderness. Do this quietly and thoughtfully for a moment before you continue reading.

Now you are beginning to know TappyBear. Now you have been fully introduced to him and can see why he is not just a toy — not even just a therapeutic stuffed animal. TappyBear is a metaphor for YOU. He is an ever-present reminder of all that is inside of you or in anyone else. He reminds you of how well *you* can really listen when you want to, how deeply and unconditionally you can love, how loyal you can be in your heart, and how beautiful and miraculous you are inside. He shows you how much power you possess and how much compassion lives in your every cell. He reminds you of how much you have to give to others. But most of all, he taps YOU on the nose and reminds you just how much of all that is wonderful you have to give to yourself.

Let me give you an example of Tappy's "magic power." It is an account written by one of the editors of this book, Ginny Grimsley, about her 7-year old daughter, Eliot, and her TappyBear.

———————————

In Ginny's words:

If there were such as thing as "Stuffed Animal Addicts Anonymous," Eliot, bless her, would be the first to raise her hand in a meeting and take the podium. All of her life, she has asked for nothing else, claiming that just THAT kitty or THIS elephant would be all she would ever want as long as she lived. However, once she receives one, she spends perhaps 24 hours smitten, then moves on. Her tendency to sometimes abandon things once the newness wears off is one of the many things that have made her response to Tappy so startling. Right from the start, Eliot and Tappy were tight. Where Eliot went, Tappy went — he was the first to achieve such a rank.

Just over a month ago, at this writing, I had never heard of EFT (*Emotional Freedom Techniques*) or TappyBear. Dr. Carrington had asked me to assist her with the editing of this guidebook for you, and when she so kindly told me that she would be sending my family a TappyBear, I have to admit I thought, "Oh my stars! Another stuffed animal! Whoa!" (If I could only impress upon you the square footage in my home dedicated to bean-filled representations of every species on the planet, you probably *still* would not believe the overall mass of fake fur in our home). But, since a new stuffed animal would be arriving — and one that I was highly interested in — I figured that Eliot should be part of that excitement. So I told her that, even though *I* would be working with Tappy, he could be hers and he would be arriving soon. She couldn't wait and came home from school every day asking if Tappy had arrived.

Several days later, there was his box on my front porch. I was curious to see all of his little tapping buttons. I wanted to know what all the hullabaloo was about. But I waited for Eliot.

When she bolted in the door from her school day, she saw the box on the dining room table and squealed, "He's HERE!" Right away, she grabbed her little scissors to slice the tape. A few struggles here and there, and then she closed her eyes, plunged her arms into the box and pulled him out. Holding him up to her face, she opened her eyes. What astonished me was that there was no "response" at all. She didn't squeal. She didn't smile. She just stared at him for a long time.

I couldn't understand this at first; this was not at all her signature response to anything that came in a box with her name written on it. But for some reason, I didn't say, "Honey, are you OK? Don't you like him?" Something told me to be quiet. Later, that same "something" told me that this had been a sacred moment in Eliot's life.

Then, without any change in her neutral expression, she pulled the bear to her chest, put her arms tight around him and rested her cheek on his head. Without looking at me, she turned and they walked together to her room.

She closed the door. When it was time for dinner, she joined us again, holding tight to Tappy's paw. She was smiling. Something had changed within her.

Eliot is a child who struggles a great deal with the emotional demands of her heart. This heart of hers is bigger than the body that carries it, but, her mind bullies that heart to such an extent that very few of us get a real glimpse of its secret hiding place. If you're not looking closely, you might mistake her for the Grinch, but it is only that she loves (and hurts) so deeply — with such intensity — that she can sometimes be oppressive and overwhelmingly attached. She knows how to cut to the quick with her words, and she will cut anyone who crosses "her" territory — anyone who interacts with her beloved people or things.

Her true love is her best friend Brooke. At school, Eliot has become known (according to her) as the meanest kid in the class because she fights (verbally) with other kids over her friend who — in Eliot's world — belongs to her alone. But Eliot hurts just as deeply as she loves, and because she holds her cards tight to her chest, that hurt is often expressed as anger instead of tears. And, of course, the behavior that results from anger — and the reaction to it from others — then hurts her even more. As her mother, my heart often aches for hers.

As I watched her with Tappy on this day that he came to us, I wondered if perhaps there was something his presence could do for her, but I had no idea where that thought came from.

Before bed that night, Eliot asked me why Tappy had button-like round spots on his body. I thought about what to say — I still didn't know much about EFT. I said, "Well, Tappy is a helper bear. When a child is sad, afraid, hurt, angry — anything that feels yucky — they can hold Tappy and tap on the buttons in a certain way that's called 'EFT' — that's short for *'Emotional Freedom Techniques'* — and this makes them feel better. Just like the name *'Emotional Freedom Techniques,'* the tapping — and Tappy — frees the bad feelings and lets them leave you, so you feel better." And I told her about how Tappy has been helping children in Mexico who have cancer and are in the hospital away from their families (see Chapter 4 for more on this important project).

Unlike the highly inquisitive Eliot I am used to, she asked no further questions. She just looked into Tappy's eyes and said, "Tappy, I'm so glad that you came here to be with me, too."

And, indeed, that is what happened — Tappy was there for her in a special way.

The next day, Eliot took Tappy to school with her and wanted to give a "presentation" to her class about him. I was hesitant because many times Eliot has presented prized "things" (almost always stuffed toys), and this has caused much drama and angst due to some other child wanting to hold or touch the toy. NO ONE touches Eliot's things. It's practically a school rule. But, again, something told me that it would be OK this time.

When I picked her up from school that afternoon, Eliot jumped into the car holding Tappy in a firm little hand: "Mommy! Tappy was GREAT in the presentation! All the kids wanted to hold him, hug him, and pet him! They asked about his buttons and everything! I told them that he was a helper bear and that you tap on the buttons to make you feel better. Mrs. Hills asked how that happened, and I told them the tapping thing was called 'EFT' or *Emotional Freedom Techniques.*' Louis said that he needed to hold Tappy because he needed some emotional freedom because he doesn't get to stay up as late as he wants. Mom, I don't think he knows what 'emotional' means, but I let him hold Tappy anyway, and he did feel better. Tappy is MAGIC!"

Let me stress again: NO ONE touches Eliot's stuff. And no one touches Eliot either. She is the type of person who has many acquaintances but very few deep friendships. Though it appears that she chooses this life, I know better. She has "slipped" a few times and told me that she wishes some child or other would be her friend. But Eliot turns away for fear of being hurt. And by doing so she comes across as "tough" and "independent." But she also comes across as cold, when, in actuality, she's extremely warm.

And when I say, "no one touches her stuff," I could put special emphasis on Louis. For it was with little Louis that Eliot fought daily over the attentions of "her" Brooke. "I hate Louis!" was her everyday mantra. Yet she allowed him to hold Tappy!

So what I think happened here, on the day Eliot took Tappy to school, was that she took the *real* Eliot to school. Perhaps it was because she knew Tappy was a helper bear. Perhaps she was just in good spirits that day. Perhaps it was a miracle... But for whatever reason, Tappy changed Eliot's accustomed behavior, her spirit, and her energy that day — and the result was wondrous.

Tappy worked for Eliot in that when she let go of him and handed him to the child closest to her in the circle, she seemed to let go of *her* fear of being hurt. Suddenly she trusted that he would be "safe" as he was passed from child to child. And when her heart decided to trust, she watched what can happen when you open yourself up — when you truly let go of fear. She saw that the children were gentle with Tappy and interested in him. She saw that they loved him and shared him freely. She saw that, in the end, he came right back to her — whole and even more wonderful than before. *What she had feared had not occurred.*

Could it be, then, that if she lets herself share who she is — even though she's afraid — that she will come back to herself just the same and even better? She had used Tappy, without knowing it, to go through what she could not. She used Tappy as a way of modeling what it looked like to be truly herself. She saw what *she* would look like if she showed the world the good that she holds inside. She saw that this was a powerful thing to do.

In the same way, she used Tappy as a tool to unlock the compassion that she struggles to show to others. She said to me: "Mommy, I hurt Brooke's feelings by accident today. I didn't mean to. She started to cry. So I went to my cubby and got Tappy. I told her to tap the button on top of his head — that it would make her feel better. And, you know what? It did! She stopped crying, and she even started laughing! I swear, I love that bear!"

As I said, Brooke has been Eliot's true love (and vice versa) since they were four years old. Theirs is one of the deepest loves I've ever seen between two people. Brooke is gentle, sweet and sensitive, while Eliot appears to be her direct opposite. However, they are very much the same in that their hearts are very deep — they feel so much. They just have opposite ways of showing the same feelings. Eliot's reactions are not as "acceptable" as Brooke's. When hurt exists between them, Brooke cries whereas Eliot gets ticked off and yells, "You deserved it!" (They were MADE for each other!) But when Brooke cries, Eliot has very rarely gone to her to apologize or make it better, even though I can always tell that she wants to. Brooke's pain tortures Eliot. And it's painful to watch Eliot deny herself what she wants to do — soothe her friend — because of fear.

TappyBear showed Eliot how to comfort Brooke. Just by seeing TappyBear — a completely open being — saying (in effect), "Here is the top of my head. You can tap on it if it makes you feel better. I am your friend, and I am here for just *you in your pain*." Eliot saw what her *own* compassion looks like, what it does for others and what it can do for her. Tappy showed Eliot what SHE would look like if she let her true heart speak for itself.

What Ginny has written about her daughter Eliot substantiates what I said before about TappyBear being a representation of the real you — the good inside of you that we were all born with. In my opinion, TappyBear, in this sense, is magical.

I don't use the word "magic" lightly here. What happened between Ginny's little daughter and Tappy, even though it may seem small, was, in a sense, in the realm of real-life "magic."

Magic, I believe, is what happens when the deepest, most open, most tender and true parts of ourselves — our souls, if you will — are able to emerge from hiding, become manifest in the outside world, and thereby change us forever. These magical moments in our lives can change not only ourselves, but everyone around us.

In my experience with TappyBear, he evokes this sort of experience. He is not "magic" itself — he is simply the open, fearless gaze, the listening ears, the warm soft tummy, the wide arms that say, "Look how perfect you are! When you look at me, you see yourself. What you believe I can do, *you* can do. So let's put you out there as you are and let you shine! Time's a wastin'!" And then it is YOU who creates the magic that we call "change."

So take a good, long, loving look at yourself as you receive this little bear. You can create magic within yourself and within others when you let yourself listen without distraction, hold firm the eyes of another who needs you, open your mind, heart, spirit, and arms without fear. When you live for those moments in which you serve yourself and others with the biggest of hearts, you are truly… you.

So, here in your hands is a friendly being who will stroll along with you and remind you, when you need reminding, that you — just as you are — are magical.

This can, and will, change everything.

Chapter 2

Tappy's Origins

The therapeutic stuffed toy known as "TappyBear" was created through the inspiration of an 11-year-old girl, Christina Schilling. Fittingly and perfectly, Tappy was made — as all truly good things are — through the mind of a child; for no matter the size or age of that person's body, it is those who maintain the spirit of child-like wonder and play who truly create what is pure in its service.

Christina, helping a neighbor, had been babysitting a five-year old boy who had a severe and embarrassing problem that no one could understand or remedy. He was inadvertently wetting himself repeatedly during the day, and since his pediatrician could find nothing physically wrong with him, his parents were told he had a developmental problem that was "most likely related to stress." However, no one had been able to determine just what that "stress" might be.

As it happened, Christina's father, Till Shilling, had recently returned from a workshop where he had learned a new, "exciting and groundbreaking" stress management technique known as *EFT: Emotional Freedom Techniques.* As he explained it to his family, it was a calming method based on the ancient art of acupuncture. But, instead of needles, EFT used just a light tapping of the fingertips.

Till had been so enthusiastic about EFT that he immediately taught it to his wife and two young daughters. At first, the girls rolled their eyes in mockery of this method because the tapping seemed a bit "weird." However, when they found that it was useful for some of their friends, they began using it themselves and were surprised at the positive results they were getting for the relief of test anxiety, for improving their athletic performance, and for strengthening and maintaining peaceful relationships with their chums — along with a whole host of other benefits.

So, as Christina watched her little charge withdraw more and more due to his condition, she puzzled over how to help him. Then it occurred to her to try EFT with him. But that presented a problem. She knew that a five-year old wouldn't take to sitting still and repeating phrases just because he was told to do so. Then she had a sudden inspiration about how to get around this problem. She decided to use one of her old teddy bears, the most beat up of the lot, and sew buttons on it to indicate where the EFT tapping spots were.

Since she is a child who is always involved in creative handiwork and loves to make handmade gifts for people (no store-bought things ever!), she created a quite presentable "EFT Bear" from her old teddy — complete with proper tapping points. She then set about teaching the little boy a "tapping game" using the bear she'd made. She asked him to find the "secret spots" on the bear (indicated by the buttons hidden in the fur) and tap on

13

them while repeating out loud with great emphasis, "Even though I wet my pants and that's *embarrassing*, I'm still a great kid!"— and other phrases to that effect.

The game was very simple, but challenging enough to hold his attention. The only rule was that he had to find all the tapping spots — he would have to find *all* of them in the fur of the bear. The little boy got into the spirit of the game immediately and began squealing with delight as he yelled out the phrases that Christina asked him to repeat. He played this EFT game until he was happily exhausted, and whenever Christina babysat for him, she always brought the bear.

Very quickly, the mother of Christina's charge noticed an unusual occurrence — her son didn't wet his pants as frequently. Within a week, to her astonishment, the problem stopped altogether. The little boy now had complete control of his bladder and, to boot, was delighted with the "tapping game."

But the story doesn't stop there. Christina's father had happened to enter the room when Christina was leading this child in the tapping game. He looked at the old beat-up bear with the buttons she had sewed on him, saw how beautifully the boy was responding to the game, and realized that his daughter had inadvertently hit upon a new way of introducing the remarkable healing technique known as EFT to children everywhere — to use for all kinds of problems. It was at that moment that "TappyBear"— the therapeutic stuffed animal that is now created especially for this purpose — came into being.

The TappyBear project now became a family adventure. Till took Christina and her younger sister Anna to a number of toy stores where they examined all of the stuffed bears on the premises and took photos of them. Later, looking at the photos, they selected the special features they thought "TappyBear" should have. This was a task that involved much discussion.

Should his ears be stiff or floppy? Christina's mother thought the ears should be stiff and face straight forward to indicate that Tappy was listening to the child's every word. The girls agreed heartily.

What color eyes should he have? Both girls thought he have the same color eyes as a beloved mongrel dog that they had rescued from the pound several years before. When this dog had come to live with them, both children had gasped when they saw his eyes. "Look! He has the eyes of an angel" Christina had cried out. Accordingly, the family selected deep blue, thoughtful "understanding" eyes for TappyBear.

How big should he be? This was important because they wanted him to be big enough to be "really huggable." They chose a size of about 15 inches in height when seated.

How soft and pliable should he be? The girls wanted him to be a sturdy, comforting presence, but he should also be soft enough to be really cuddly.

Should he have just the stumps of feet that most stuffed bears have, or should he have real bear-like feet? The girls wanted real looking bear feet with delineated toes, and so they created Tappy's great paws.

Typically teddy bears have very flat small noses — almost no noses at all. The girls wanted Tappy to have a *real* nose, a bear snout that would make him seem alive.

They chose his present prominent white nose.

Now there remained the question of a trademark. What could that be? This last question was answered when the family visited an Indian reservation in Canada where they watched a ritual dance performed by members of the tribe. The medicine man who led the dance wore a bearskin, complete with the bear's head, over his own. Nine-year old Anna, the resident artist of the family, went up to him fearlessly and asked, "Mister? Where did you get that costume?" The medicine man then crouched down before her so that his eyes were level with her own, and answered seriously, "The bear is a very powerful animal; it affords protection to everyone, including little girls like you. That is why I wear his skin."

Anna thanked him, and when the family returned home she pulled out her many painting and drawing supplies and her endless reams of paper and began sketching an idea that had come to her as a result of the visit to Canada. It was of a great big strong bear paw upon which was superimposed the innocent and trusting hand of a little child. The family made some suggestions and moved the positioning of the child's hand several times, but the picture was essentially little Anna's creation and is today the trademark that one sees embroidered on the sole of one of Tappy's feet.

Then came the final step. Till had to find an appropriate manufacturer for Tappy. He had been an executive with a large pharmaceutical company, and it had been his job to negotiate shipments of products from China and other countries. He knew well the respectful attitude one needs to have when conducting such negotiations.

But it was not easy to find a manufacturer who was willing to take on the job of making TappyBear. Typically, overseas manufacturers will accept nothing smaller than an order for 25,000 units at a time. However, Till finally located one factory in China that agreed to make a semi-hand-assembled TappyBear, and thereby no two bears would be exactly alike.

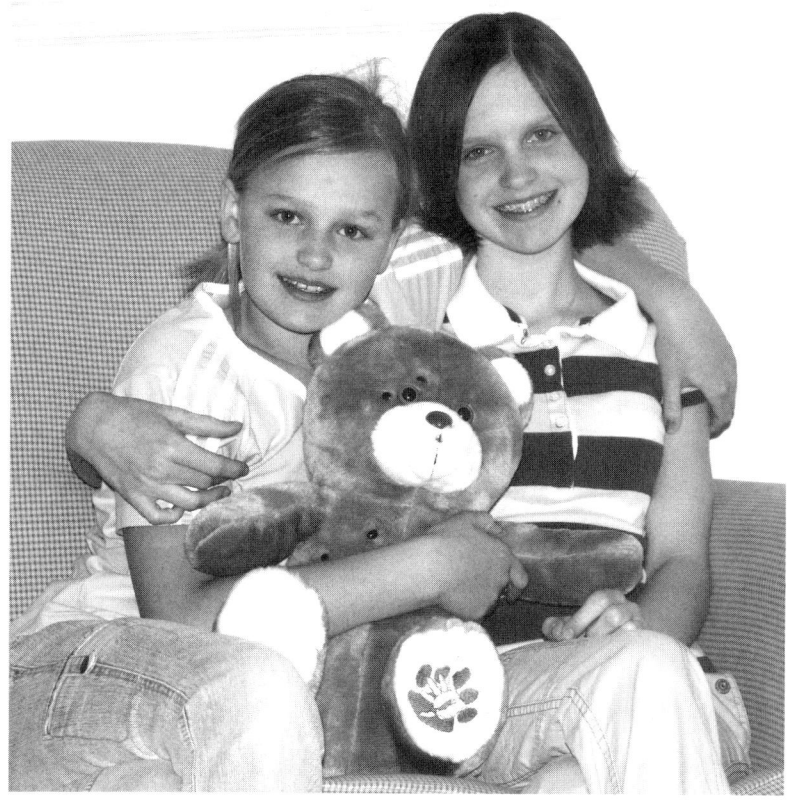

Inventors Anna (left) and Christina (right) Schilling at the time when TappyBear came into being.

17

And so it is a rare and unusual bear toy, created out of love and caring and a spirit of sharing, that is personified in TappyBear today. Tappy is bringing healing and love to many children, and to an increasingly large number of adults, in many parts of the world. It seems almost as though he has come to the world to spread a message of simple kindness, and sincere caring. Those of us who work with Tappy are devoted to him.

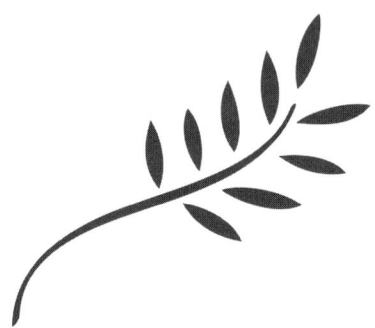

Chapter 3

How Tappy Works with Children

As you will see, Tappy, in his special way, "unwraps" the gift of delight in that he appears as a teddy bear, but his true gift is the healing process that can come through EFT. The following reports are meant to give you guidance and inspiration as you use your creative, intuitive spirit to find your *own* way with Tappy. Tappy has a sacred occupation, and your role now is simply to put him into the arms of a child and listen with alert ears to his or her fears, needs and joys. Listen, be amazed, and use all of your intuition to act upon whatever message Tappy brings you.

First, I'll begin with the "call to arms." Before the wonderful invention of TappyBear, Gary Craig, the founder of *EFT: Emotional Freedom Techniques*, wrote the following article for his newsletter urging a strong mission for parents, teachers, therapists and practitioners who use EFT to focus their attention on serving the needs of our children.

In our world community, the possibilities for healing with EFT are vast, and to create a well world, we must begin by allowing our children access to the power to heal. Now that TappyBear has entered the picture and become a "tapping" helper, what Gary envisions for every child, and for the world, is that much of what was before was impossible is now possible when EFT (in many instances delivered through TappyBear) becomes a part of this loving process of teaching and healing children.

In his statement, now posted on www.emofree.com, Gary speaks of the use of EFT for children:

"(With EFT)... together we can do something very special for our children.

When I say our children I don't just mean those who grow up in our individual households and carry around our last names. I mean the children of the world — everyone's children. I'm talking about the little folks of today who become the big folks of tomorrow and influence the direction of this planet.

I was a little kid once. So were you. Were you afraid of the Boogey Man at night like I was? Did you bite your fingernails like I did? I was never abused in any manner but maybe you were? What's it like to carry that into adulthood? Do you have fears, guilt and "limits" now because of unresolved abuse of long ago? What about those who had dyslexia or other learning disabilities? Were they ridiculed as children? Put down? Held back in school? Told they weren't very smart? Believed it? And, what's worse, STILL believe it?

Do some of our children have anger at how they are treated? Do they carry that into adulthood and act it out? How many of our children feel they "don't belong" because they aren't smart enough, rich enough, pretty enough or don't know the right people? Do drugs make them feel better about themselves?

Our childhood experiences tend to establish the avenues we take through life. Some of us spend our lives stalled on Anxiety Avenue or Woe-Is-Me Way while others move freely along Success Street, Heaven's Highway and Love's Lane. Do you suppose our unresolved fears, traumas, guilt and other baggage-like emotions from childhood have any influence on which freeways we frequent?

Of course they do. Our childhood experiences are written on our emotional walls and, depending on their quality, they become either "stop signs" or "green lights" as we move through life. Further, they have a way of reinforcing themselves and growing larger over time. A child made to feel stupid will see the world through "stupid eyes" and gather continuing evidence for his/her stupidity. By contrast, a child who is made to feel like a wonder child will see the world through confident eyes and gather evidence for his/her wondrous nature.

So what is this special thing I said earlier that we could do together for our children? I'll get to that in a moment but first, let's explore what you might do on your own. Perhaps you could use EFT in a child's behalf to resolve an anger issue or dissipate a firmly held fear. Would that help point the child down a new freeway? Sure! Could you eliminate some learning disabilities, relieve headaches and nightmares or get rid of some tendencies to stutter? Sure again! There is much that you can do for our children and each time you do so you replace friction in their lives with a form of freedom. Shifts like this during childhood have a way of echoing into adulthood. They gather evidence to reinforce themselves and thus magnify a few well played loving notes into a symphony.

You even feel good about yourself in the process. Nobody loses in this effort. It's an everybody wins deal. For those looking for a mission, here's a clear candidate. Do you hear Mission Music in this? I hope so — for your sake as well as for the sake of the children."

Helping Your Child *and* Yourself With EFT

It's important to remember that Tappy teaches a form of EFT for children, but Tappy can also work as a reminder to parents to take care of themselves as they care for their little ones. After all, wellbeing for children begins with the wellbeing of their parents. EFT has powerful stress-relieving benefits, which are priceless when one is a parent. It is a valuable tool in calming yourself before bringing the gift of EFT to your child. In fact, as you'll see in Chapter 5, Till Schilling, the father of Christina Schilling, who helped create the original TappyBear, usually recommends introducing Tappy to the adult first, and then the child. Tappy is a good teacher of peace and relaxation during stressful situations for both you and your children. An account by Steve Wells, a leading EFT psychologist from Australia, can gives insight into how to use EFT when dealing with children who are "getting on your last nerve." He wrote the following article before there was a TappyBear, but Tappy can help the process even more.

"Using EFT with your own children can be a most rewarding experience. It can also be extremely frustrating. Here are a couple of things I have learned from using EFT with my own children.

1) You need to do the tapping on yourself first.

If it isn't working, I would suggest this is the first place you should look, particularly with younger children. They tend to be intimately tied to your own emotional state to determine how they are going to feel. Remember, emotions get transferred between people when we interact, and children are often like tuning forks for our emotional states.

Case in point. One night my son Joshua, age 6, was frightened to go into his room alone telling me he was scared there might be ghosts in there. After explaining that there were no ghosts, and that his light was still on — traditional linear parental logic — he still refused. I told him I would do "the tapping" on this for him to help him to be less afraid. He replied that the tapping would not work (I've found the Apex phenomena is rife even with young children!).

I have tended to ignore such protests in the past as he has had excellent results from EFT even while protesting, *"this won't work"*. I proceeded to rub on his sore spot and say, *"Even though you're scared of ghosts, you're still a good kid."* Following several rounds and no reduction in fear I, in my frustration, implemented plan B: Exposure treatment —*"Feel the fear and do it anyway kid"*!

What followed was a very upset little boy who went to his room under extreme sufferance, which was followed by another performance when going to the bathroom to brush his teeth, and still more crying and upset over going to the toilet. Following this, and with me feeling like a total chump for forcing him to suffer so, I took a moment out to think and do some tapping on myself. Then, having produced a little necessary distance, I sat down on the bed with him and started to talk about what was scaring him.

As I was now no longer anxious about his anxiety (or as frustrated with it), I found I was available to listen to him more fully — and target the treatment towards his specific fears — and he was surprisingly more receptive to the EFT as well. He told me about a segment in a TV program with an airship full of ghosts. Not only the images but also what was said on the program had upset him. I asked if he would be able to focus on that while we did the tapping and he agreed.

As he did so, I was able to realize that the slight distance I now had was crucial to getting this to work for him. I needed to be free of my own negative emotional states ABOUT his problem, in order to work with him ON his problem. Prior to this my emotions were clouding my responsibility — and even being transferred to him, short-circuiting our work together.

I believe if we *anxiously* tap with someone or on someone we greatly lessen our chances of a positive result — this is why I always tap along with my clients. I don't want my own state to interfere with their healing. Anyway, the conclusion to this story is that we were then able to proceed through several aspects, with me being respectful enough of my son to ask him at each point *"What should we call that?"* when we identified aspects to tap on, involving him more fully in the process. Five rounds later and he's off to sleep. Problem solved — at least for now!

My advice to other parents and to therapists: Always, always, always tap on yourself. I have experienced numerous situations where this has made all the difference."

Steve then goes on to tell us:

2) Treat yourself for the things your children do that upset you.

When my daughter was born, her particularly loud cry and inbuilt persistence had a significant negative effect on me. I found it mightily stressful to deal with her at these times of auditory assault.

One day while changing her nappy, with her screaming and me getting upset, I realized I needed to do some tapping on this. A few rounds of tapping on her cry and I suddenly became aware of the wide variety of different cries she actually produced. Previously they were all the same — loud and intensely upsetting for me. Now I realized that some cries were due to real pain, some were due to frustration, some were from her simply wanting a little love and affection, etc, etc. Previously, they all translated to me as intense pain. And that was painful for me to cope with so I wanted to immediately jump in and settle her down. Especially when a particularly tired girl could take up to an hour to settle herself down to sleep.

After tapping on myself over her cry, I was able to realize that not all her cries required an immediate response, or the same type of response, or even any response at all on occasions. And I began to feel good about my little girl again. I wish I could say she stopped yelling and screaming. I can report that now almost two years later she does settle more quickly. But the empowerment of being able to "stand in the heat" was significant for a father who never would have been able to cope with this without the tapping."

EFT Can Teach Compassion

One of the most extraordinary gifts that EFT gives to children (and grown-ups as well) is an open and loving way to heal others. As parents, when using EFT as a tool for relieving your child's pain, you open up, quite unexpectedly at times, a door for them to become healers themselves. Compassion is a trait we all hope to foster in our children, yet it is sometimes difficult to "teach" them how to express this natural, human tendency. *Speaking* to them about being compassionate toward others can be frustrating and ineffective. We speak the word "share" to them again and again when they are little, and flinch to see them become tiny dictators over every toy in the room.

The only real way to convey the importance of compassion is to model it. As parents, we do this as we constantly give love and understanding to our children. EFT and Tappy offer a tangible new way to show them what it means to help and serve others. As you use EFT and Tappy with your children, the relief of pain they experience quickly teaches them how amazing it feels to be helped in this manner when they themselves are in dire need. Naturally, they will then want to heal others in need as well.

Ginny Grimsley's story about her daughter Eliot's sudden shift toward wanting to help and heal her friends is a good example of this. Eliot was 7-years old when she discovered Tappy and EFT, and although her story exemplifies how children learn to heal others through EFT and Tappy in lovely ways, the next story is almost shocking because it shows that even an 18-month-old child can learn to act as Eliot did.

Diane Keast wrote a letter to Gary Craig that was published in emofree.com concerning her daughter Kelsea (name changed) who, when 18 months old, suffered extreme teething pain. This pain was so intense that Kelsea could not eat and reverted back to the bottle after having been weaned for over six months. Diane used pain relievers for some time, but Kelsea still struggled with sleep, crankiness, and eating problems.

One day it occurred to Diane to use EFT with Kelsea but found that her daughter didn't like to be tapped. So, instead, Diane used a gentle, circular movement on the EFT points. This calmed Kelsea considerably, much to everyone's relief, and when she got used to the tapping points being touched, then her mother began using the tapping. From that point on, Kelsea would come to Diane to be tapped when she was upset or in pain.

Diane's story doesn't stop here however. The reaches of EFT go beyond relieving your child's pain or teaching them how to relieve their own. As Diane describes Kelsea's behavior with another child, it's clear that EFT has the power to inspire compassion and the wish to heal others, even among the smallest of us. Her mother writes:

"Recently Kelsea was playing with a little boy her age who didn't want to share with her. Every time she would try to take a toy, he would squeal at

28

the top of his lungs and start to cry. Each time this happened, my daughter would reach over and gently tap the top of his head, and he would stop. She was very gentle and he seemed to enjoy it.

This went on all night. Whenever he started to cry about her sharing the toys she would tap him gently on the top of his head. She tapped him again and again until she had tapped him into a calm state, and he felt OK about sharing with her. We are so thrilled to be able to offer our daughter such a positive tool."

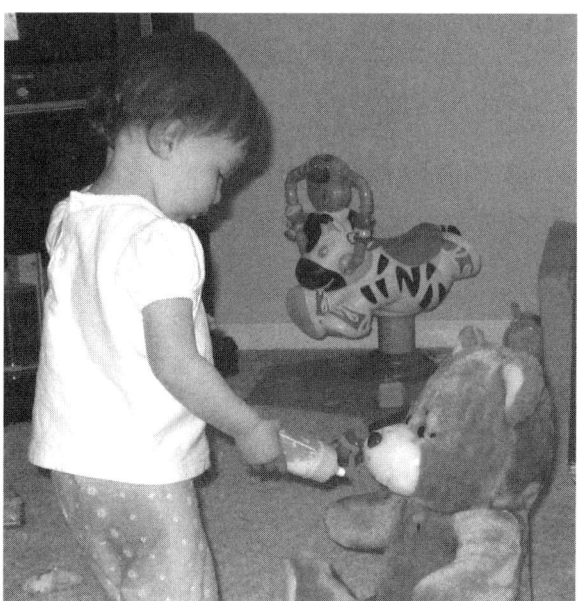

17 month old Caroline loves to give Tappy his bottle.

Kids Help Themselves by Helping Tappy

I think you will find much of interest in this next story for many reasons. EFT Practitioner, Dr. Kiya Immergluck, a Licensed Clinical Counselor, relates a real-life story that gives us a chance to really see TappyBear at work. She shows us how quickly a shy little boy responded when she helped him place his fears into Tappy so that the child could "heal" Tappy, and thus himself. This is one of the most compelling ways to allow Tappy to do his magic — especially for a younger child in a therapeutic setting.

"Recently, I had the privilege of teaching EFT to a number of pre-school children and their mothers. In each case, the Mom had heard about EFT and specifically, TappyBear, a cuddly teddy bear with buttons to represent the basic tapping points. In one particular case, "Mrs. Jones" called me on a Sunday asking for an emergency session that same day.

Her son Joey is 5 years old and painfully shy. It was very difficult to convince him to go to kindergarten at the beginning of the year, but after a two-week vacation, he absolutely refused to go back. I made a house call and brought a TappyBear for Joey. I went to the house with low expectations. I surrogate-tapped for Joey (this is tapping on one's own EFT points with the intention of helping another person), and prayed too, on my way:

Even though I don't like talking to strangers, I'm a great kid.

Even though I'm scared to go back to school, I'm a great kid.

Even though I'm scared to talk to anyone, I'm a great kid.

When I arrived, Mrs. Jones warned me that Joey just cried when she explained that *"a lady is coming to play with you with a teddy bear."* He was interested in the bear, but wanted nothing to do with *the lady.* He declared to his Mom, *I won't talk to her — I won't even look at her!*

I walked into the living room and saw a tiny little boy huddled into the cushions of the couch with his face turned away. I came in very quietly and whispered, *TappyBear is scared… can you help him?* What happened next seemed nothing short of a miracle to me and to Joey's Mom. I was prepared to spend an hour helping Joey feel safe enough to look at me and maybe say *hello* to me. Instead, Joey jumped off the couch, came right over and gently cuddled TappyBear.

I brought along a story about TappyBear and began reading it to Joey as a way to teach him the tapping points. My theory is that most very young children love to be *helpers* and would enjoy helping TappyBear get over his fears.

Whenever the story suggested that Joey tap on the bear and say, *I'm a great bear*, Joey spontaneously began tapping on himself *and* the bear saying,

31

I'm a great kid AND I'm a great bear! By the time we got done with the story, Joey was comfortable tapping on the bear and on himself. He was also very comfortable talking with me!

I said at the end of the story, *You know, TappyBear is also scared to go to school. Do you think we could help him?* Joey was very eager to help TappyBear again, and when I asked him what Tappy was afraid of, he told me many very specific complaints that *TappyBear* had:

> *TappyBear is scared that he can't do the work...*
>
> *TappyBear is scared that he can't talk to the other kids...*
>
> *TappyBear doesn't like that the school day is too long...*

So, Joey verbalized exactly what issues he needed to tap on. Next, I taught Joey to hold his arms outstretched to show that TappyBear was very, very upset. Then, I showed him how to bring his hands closer and closer together to show that Tappy was getting less and less scared. Finally, I showed him how to have his palms touch (like hands in prayer) to indicate that the fears were completely gone.

By the end of the session, Joey collapsed all of Tappy's fears about school, and even added in some extra fears about creepy, crawly bugs. The session went very well and Joey was smiling and shook my hand when I left.

Mrs. Jones reported that Joey wasn't thrilled to go to school the next day, but the extreme fears were definitely greatly reduced. Joey loves his TappyBear and enjoys having Tappy's story read to him again and again! TappyBear is a wonderful tool for teaching EFT to young children, and it is also a terrific icebreaker with shy and non-communicative children."

Using TappyBear with *Teens*?

When we think of introducing a young child to EFT and TappyBear, the vision is quite easy to conjure up. Young children, after all, love stuffed animals and are more open to new ideas and situations. It's harder to imagine presenting TappyBear to an adolescent. You might imagine a great deal of eye-rolling and out-right rejection. It's important to remember, however, that it is not essential that the child become a "believer" in the benefit of tapping for them to receive benefits as they tap — or as you tap for them. TappyBear, even with adolescents (who really are still children underneath), can often break the stone wall that they put up when they are suffering.

Till Schilling, in the following letter that was first posted in www.emofree.com, relates a fascinating example of just how well Tappy can work with teenagers. Granted, the Schillings have used EFT as a source of family healing for many years, but Till's tale shows that while a teenager can "buck" what they've always trusted and lash out at it, patience and persistence (and a bit of TappyBear) can turn things around. Till writes:

"A while ago, I picked my daughter (11) up from school. As she got in the car, she started very intensely voicing her frustration about several disciplinary processes. How unfair it was that good kids had to pay for the misbehavior of a few troublemakers, etc. So intense was her reaction that everyone in her path, including me, was a victim of her anger tsunami. This was totally atypical of her, and it made me back off and observe.

After about five minutes of letting her vent her frustration, I noticed that she was caught in a downward spiral — frustration led to anger which led to more frustration and so on. In the past, I have to admit, I would have silenced her with an order. This time, inspired by an article I read about peaceful conflict resolution, I simply grabbed her TappyBear and sat down next to her on her bed.

While looking at her, I gently tapped on her Bear and simply stated some phrases in my mind as she went on venting. For her, I thought:

> *Even though I am extremely frustrated, and angry, I am a fair kid.*
>
> *Even though I am extremely frustrated, and angry, I am an awesome girl.*
>
> *Even though I am extremely frustrated, and angry, I can remain calm.*

While she was still on a roll, she saw me tapping on the Bear. At that point, she went into overdrive

— strongly dismissing EFT and ridiculing our whole EFT TappyBear effort. She stated that it was ridiculous — that there cannot be any relief simply by poking around on your body and on and on. As can be the case with anger, one starts saying things that are extremely hurtful.

I took a deep breath and kept on tapping on the Bear for her:

> *Even though I am extremely frustrated, and angry, I am a fair kid.*
>
> *Even though I am extremely frustrated, and EFT sucks, I can choose to be calm.*
>
> *Even though I am mad at what I see, and I cannot do anything about it, I can choose to react differently; I can choose to be calm.*

Generally, my non-reaction would set her off even more, but something interesting happened after three minutes of tapping time. She sat down next to me — exhausted — and, like a balloon running low on air, she went off telling me about her real frustration. She had sadness about her friend's leukemia… the war… that she does not understand religion… and then some more issues too long to write about here. It was a highly explosive emotional concoction!

What is remarkable is that there was a point during her raving at which the intensity in the pitch of her angry voice literally caved in.

35

I have to confess that I had to struggle to be able to keep calm long enough to distance myself from her anger and to concentrate on collapsing it for her. Afterward we talked and hugged for about an hour.

Remarkably, during similar situations in the past, the frustration would have ruled the rest of the day, causing all sorts of havoc on her ability to do her chores. This would invoke corresponding corrective measures from us, resulting in totally unnecessary escalation. Instead, her chores were not only finished on time, but I was also helped in the kitchen with cleanup with no extra motivation."

As you can see from these stories, TappyBear is a true helper, and, as a tool for EFT, he goes a long way toward fulfilling the vision set forth in Gary Craig's message at the start of this chapter.

I have shared the above stories to give you some idea of how Tappy and EFT have been used with children of various ages. I hope these accounts will inspire you as you begin this journey with TappyBear. The next chapter will show you that this delightful stuffed companion can also be used to aid healing in medical settings with serious health conditions. And if you would like to read more about Tappy and his amazing effects on children, please visit www.tappybear.com.

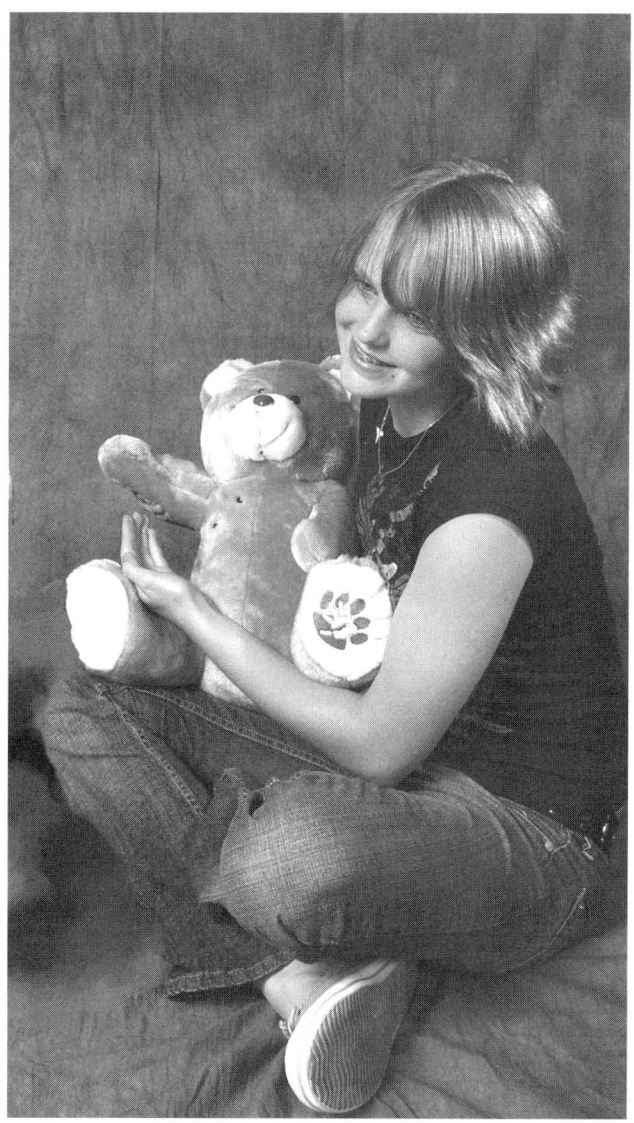

A teenager taps contentedly on the Bear's Karate Chop Spot.

Chapter 4

Using TappyBear in a Medical Setting

Though EFT is short for *Emotional Freedom Techniques*, its uses are certainly not limited to emotional issues. Parents all over the world are beginning to joyfully discover the benefits tapping can produce when used with children who are sick, injured and suffering from a wide range of physical ailments. TappyBear now offers every family a beautiful, child-friendly "tool" to make the wonderful gift of EFT more accessible to children who are hurting.

Gary Craig, founder of EFT, is fond of saying about EFT, "Try it on everything!" This is good advice. EFT is a gentle technique that has no known adverse side effects. While it's not *guaranteed* to help every suffering child in every situation, its benefits are often so remarkable, so fast and so powerful, it begs us to answer the question: why not try it? And why not let TappyBear be your trusted helper? He can often help you reach a child when adult words and attitudes can't get through.

Here are a few stories that show how EFT, and TappyBear, can ease the suffering of children and bring them relief, hope, healing and a feeling of control in the most painful and frightening situations.

38

EFT in the ER and OR

Bobby comes from what I call an "EFT family." His mom, Anita, and her husband use EFT. Bobby, the youngest child, and his sister were brought up tapping. When Bobby was about 7 years old, he had over fifty food allergies, and his mother tapped ceaselessly for him to correct them. As a result, Bobby overcame his allergies to a remarkable degree and is no longer symptomatic.

His mother used to tap *for* Bobby and repeat the EFT phrases out loud for him (which is one good way to use EFT), but since the following events happened, she usually does not have to surrogate-tap anymore.

One day Bobby suddenly developed a severe pain in his abdomen. He could barely talk, but could only remain in bed clutching his belly. He asked for EFT, and Anita went to work using it while making an emergency call to their pediatrician. Meanwhile, she asked Bobby to "breathe through" the pain. They used the EFT phrase, "Even though I have this terrible pain, I'm an awesome kid, and I know I'm going to feel better soon."

The pain became much more bearable after the tapping, but Anita noticed that he was favoring the right side of his body when he walked. They went straight to the doctor's office, where the pediatrician pressed on his right lower abdomen. It was tender but Bobby didn't jump. It didn't look like an emergency, but the doctor decided to send him to the emergency room just to "make certain."

They arrived at the ER that morning, but it wasn't until early afternoon that the crucial blood test was done. A CT Scan followed at 7 p.m. There were many hours of waiting in the Emergency Room before it was discovered that, to everyone's surprise, Bobby's appendix had ruptured! He was prepared for emergency surgery.

How did Bobby handle the long hours of waiting in the ER in pain? Anita estimates that they tapped at least *70 percent of the time* during that long wait. She recalls that they tapped on such phrases as, "Even though I'm afraid I'm going to have to have an operation, I'm an awesome kid."

When he felt particularly powerless about what was being done to him (which was much of the time), they also used the phrase, "Even though all these things are being done to me, and I can't do anything about it, I know that Mom loves me."

Bobby expressed great fear of having his appendix out and a strong wish to keep his "busted appendix," even though he knew that by keeping it he might die. So he and his mom tapped on, "Even though if I keep my appendix I might die, I know I'll get better if I have it taken out."

Following this tapping he became much calmer, and when he met the surgeon, he liked him right away. He now decided to tap on, "Even though I don't want this operation, I'm an awesome kid, and this guy is going to get me better." Following this last round of tapping he looked straight at the surgeon and said, "OK! Let's get it done!"

Anita, who had now been joined by her husband in the emergency room, stood by, watching him in amazement. His parents were seeing a maturity in him they had never seen before. Now, instead of asking for their help in this distressing situation, he tapped on himself. The more he tapped, the more he was able to handle the situation. He no longer seemed to have anxiety about the operation itself, and, if a new issue arose that presented a fresh difficulty, he insisted they all tap on it.

When Bobby was taken to the operating room, Anita tapped continuously in the waiting room while her husband made some urgent phone calls. Her anxiety went way down, and, out of exhaustion, she had actually dozed off when the surgeon came out to greet them after the surgery. He told them that the site of the operation had been "a mess" but that the infection was so well-contained that it had not spread at all. "Never in a million years would I have dreamed we would find this kind of situation when we got in. He didn't seem sick enough for what we saw."

Anita believes that their extensive use of EFT may actually have helped to contain the infection.

The surgeon expected Bobby to be in the hospital from four to seven days, although, surprisingly, he had no fever. Post-operatively the family did even more tapping than before because Bobby was in serious pain and had to endure many needles.

They tapped a great deal for Bobby's feelings of being out of control. The result was that a quiet authority came over the child. When hospital personnel came in with medications or injections that he did not feel ready for, he would politely say to them, "I don't want to do that right now. Can I do it in an hour?" His mother doubts that she could have as effectively asserted herself under similar circumstances.

As an example of the new maturity that he was

displaying, when a nurse missed his vein twice while trying to take blood, he turned to her and calmly said, "You're not doing a very good job. Could you find someone else to do this?" So the nurse did!

Bobby then asked the hospital authorities, "What do I have to do to get these *things* (IV needles) out of my arm?" They explained to him that he needed to be able to walk down the hall, have a good bowel movement and be eating a regular diet. He then set out to make these things happen and was soon able to pass all the tests. To everyone's surprise, Bobby was released from the hospital two and a half days after surgery.

This was an amazing growth experience for Bobby. As his parents watched the way he handled himself in the hospital, they were viewing him in a new way. Anita says she would love to see every parent in the world using EFT with their children.

When, two weeks after the surgery, Bobby had to return to the ER because of a stomach virus that was complicating the final stage of his recovery (he bounced right back from this), he watched the other children in the waiting room crying and screaming in distress and said, "I sure wish all these kids could have EFT!"

TappyBear Assists a Cancer Unit

Though TappyBear is only beginning to be introduced into clinical settings, EFT Practitioner Deborah Miller has had the opportunity to use Tappy in a children's leukemia ward in Mexico. It all began when she was invited to participate in a Health Fair for Kids with Cancer. The response to Tappy was so positive, Deborah and Tappy were invited to work on the hospital unit itself.

"There is something very pleasant about seeing an adult walk into a room carrying a TappyBear," she observes. "It opens a space for me to approach the children. I ask them if they know they have "magic fingers." This usually gets a look of surprise or interest. Then I show them how they can tap on themselves or on TappyBear. Tappy helps me make contact with the children and allows me to begin tapping with them."

With the younger children, Deborah says she usually starts with a simple, positive statement, such as "You are special," "You are sweet," or "You are cute" (most of the kids have lost their hair due to chemo). She'll also use fun statements to make them laugh and positive healing statements, such as "My body knows how to heal," "I want to heal," and "I am healed," in order "to help them reset their negative beliefs about healing."

Although Deborah often does not get the chance to work with a child for more than 5-15 minutes (because there are so many of them), she also tries to help them calm their fears. As they tap, many common fears come up — fear of needles, of chemo, of the unknown, of not getting better, of pain, and fear of fear itself. "I use visualization as it often makes it easier for them to express what they are experiencing. I ask what color or shape the fear has. Many times it is black or red." She then taps to fill that place of fear with love instead. When she asks them again to describe the color of their experience, it has often changed to pink or white.

Deborah also taps with the kids to help them with physical symptoms such as vomiting, stomach pains and fever. They tap to reduce the nausea they feel during or after chemo. In most cases, she has observed, the symptoms ease considerably.

Deborah's adventures with kids in the cancer ward have only just begun. Still, there are a few friends she has made there whose stories already seem quite memorable to her. Let's look at a few of them here, in Deborah's words.

Cinthia

Deborah reports on Cinthia as follows:

She was the first child with cancer I encountered. She was, in fact, at the Fundraiser for Kids with Cancer where I did my first session with Tappy. It was held at a city park, so I met Cinthia and a few others lying on cots in a makeshift tent.

Cinthia's round face and ready smile make you warm to her immediately, and I offered to show her how to use my brand new TappyBear. She nodded enthusiastically. I showed her how to tap with Tappy and also tapped directly on her.

We tapped simple phrases such as: *I am a good kid. I'm a wonderful girl. I feel better. I want my body to heal. I am a great girl.* We tapped for about five minutes and she was all smiles and said that she felt much better.

I later met with Dr. Quero Hernández and asked him about the possibility of my working with EFT and TappyBear in the children's cancer ward. He kindly granted me free access to the ward, to the children, to the parents and even to the nurses.

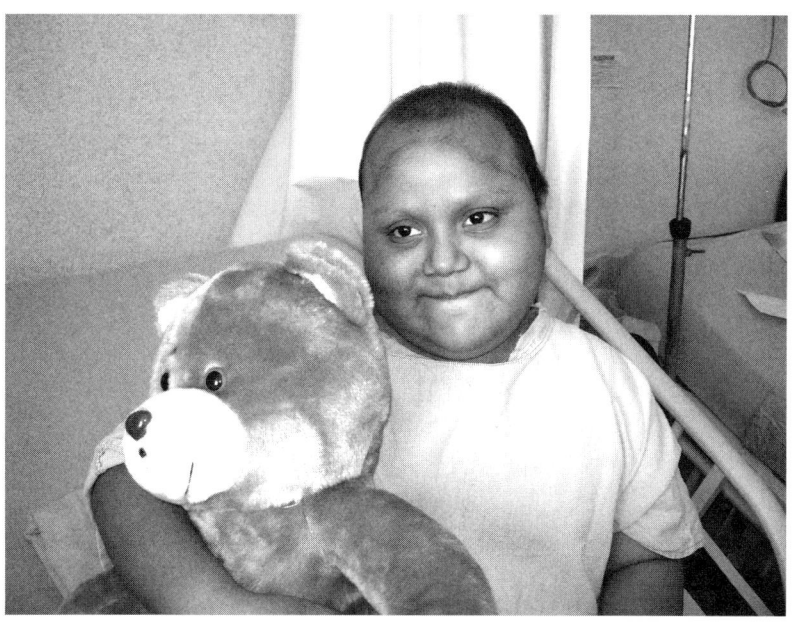

Cinthia with Tappy.

On the first day I arrived to work with the children, whom do I see but Cinthia? Though two and a half months had passed since I'd first introduced her to EFT, she remembered me right away. I asked her if she also remembered how to tap. She answered, "Oh yes, I tap all the time and I even taught my dad. He taps with me." I was pleasantly stunned. This sweet 7-year-old had taken EFT to heart because it made her feel better and then taken it another step by teaching her father. We have much to learn from children!

45

Cinthia is afraid of needles — not a good thing for a child who is being injected often and receiving chemotherapy. We started by tapping on her fears and putting "power" in her tummy. She laughed. I wanted her to understand that she was a powerful girl. She described her power as "blue." So we tapped blue power into her tummy.

The day she was due to get her next injection in her spinal column she was very frightened. She was quiet, focused on the terrible event to come. I asked her what her fear looked like. She said it was enormous and red and in her head. We tapped to make her fear smaller and smaller. In the end, we used a "needle" to pop her fear.

I have found it useful for the children to visualize the whole injection process ahead of time. In that way, we determine where they are feeling afraid. It helps them release their fear of each step of the process before they actually have the injection done.

First I had Cinthia imagine walking from her bed into the consultation room. She felt fear. We tapped: *I am afraid of going in there. It hurts when they poke me in the back. I don't like it. I'm scared. I don't like how it hurts.* Once that seemed okay, I asked her to imagine getting on the table.

Fear once again. We tapped: *I don't want to get up there. I know something that hurts is coming.* Cinthia likes angels so, while tapping, we included: *I have three angels that come with me. One is on each side of me and one is behind me. It makes me feel safe.*

Next I had her visualize the doctor coming in with the needle. That brought up lots of fear. We tapped: *I don't like that needle. It hurts me. I hate it. I don't want to cry. I don't want to be poked.* Then she made up a "good" story in her mind and tapped on that. *I relax my back and the needle goes in so easily I hardly feel it. I remember to relax and it is all over before I know it. The doctor is very gentle. I'm okay because I'm a good girl.* We reviewed the whole process until she was completely fine imagining it.

After the injection, I saw Cinthia coming out of the room with tears in her eyes. We tapped again to release the pain and to feel okay. The pain at the area of injection immediately went away. Then I asked her to tell me up to what point in the process she had been okay. She said she'd been fine until the doctor poked her. We tapped: *I was brave. I did a good job. I wasn't afraid for most of the time, just when he poked me. I don't have to be afraid anymore. I feel better faster when I tap.*

Before the next injection, we worked again at visualizing the process and releasing her fears. During the imaginary process, she was able to walk into the room and get on the table without fear. The fear came when the needle appeared. When I asked her where she felt the fear, she said in her head. It was "big, big, big and yellow." This time we tapped and imagined blowing all of that big, big, big, yellow fear into a balloon. Once it was all in there I asked her what she wanted to do with it. Again, she wanted to pop it. So we did. Most of the fear disappeared. We filled another balloon until the rest of the fear was out of her head and then we popped it again.

The following day I saw her mother who came up to me with the biggest smile you could imagine. She said the injection had gone without pain! Cinthia had been a little afraid when the process began, but then calmed herself by tapping. Cinthia told me personally that she felt no pain. She spoke about it as if it was a past issue. The doctor confirmed for me that she hadn't felt any pain. He knew from three years of experience with Cinthia how afraid she was of these treatments. He told me that she actually was singing afterwards!

Emigdio

Emigdio has leukemia. The first time I met him he was alone in the hospital bed, lying there pale, sad and without energy. When I came in with TappyBear, I saw curiosity in his eyes. Who is this woman and why is she carrying a stuffed bear? I asked him if he wanted to learn how to use his magic fingers. He nodded.

When I asked him if he felt sad or had pain, he said he didn't have any energy. Using TappyBear, we tapped about energy and his color got better as I watched! He soon sat up on his own.

The next time I saw him his color was still good and he told me he felt lots more energy. He was smiling so widely, I couldn't believe it.

"Let me ask you something, Emigdio. Do you have any fears?"

He thought for a moment, then nodded timidly.

"Can you tell me what color the fear is?"

"It doesn't have a color."

"Does it have a shape or a form?"

He thought about this for a bit, then realized it was an animal. A dog, specifically.

"Is it a ferocious dog?" I asked.

He nodded vigorously. We tapped on the fear, the dog, "the mean dog," "the black dog," "the bad dog," and then changed it into "a nice dog," "a pet dog," "a friendly dog." I asked him to close his eyes again to look at the fear that was a dog. He closed his eyes, then opened them quickly with pleasant shock on his face. He said it wasn't a bad dog, but a good dog. He was smiling from ear to ear.

The next day his dog-like fear was still gone, but he said the night before he had seen the fear as a woman, a yelling woman. We again tapped to change her from a mean, yelling woman to a nice one. It only took a minute or two. Another layer of his fear had appeared and, this time, quickly disappeared. I reminded him to tap on himself whenever he felt fear.

The following day, the nurse reported to me that Emigdio had excitedly told her about how we had used TappyBear to get rid of his fears.

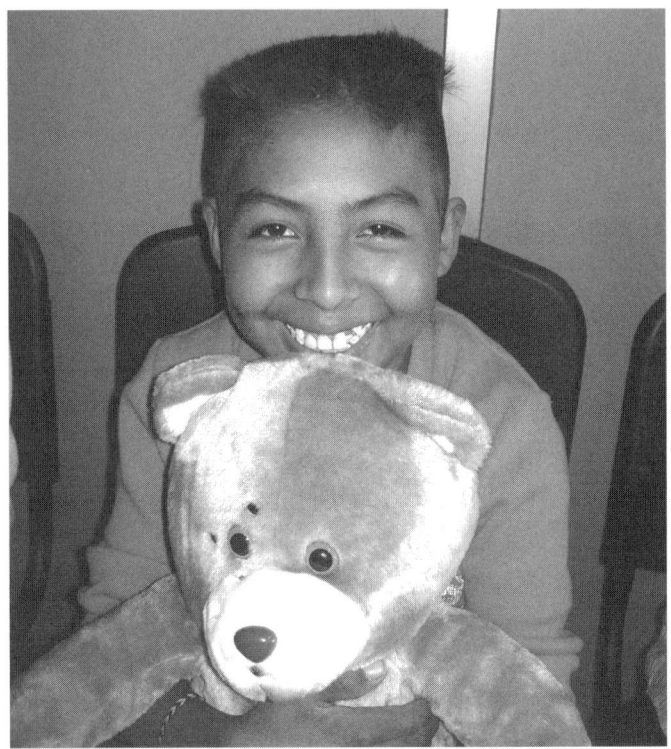

Emigdio with Tappy.

50

A few weeks later, Emigdio was in ICU with an intestinal infection. He told me the infection was green, an ugly green. We used TappyBear to release his image of his disease. As we tapped he decided to burn it. It took a while but then it was gone. We put healing "energy" in its place.

Now that I knew him a little better, I decided to venture, "Do you remember when you first got sick, Emigdio?" And something remarkable came up.

Without a moment's pause, he said, "three years ago when my little brother got sick." *That* fear, he said, was like "*lots* of bad dogs." We tapped to release those fears/bad dogs. I asked him if there was anything else. There was.

"I was scared for my little brother so I promised to get sick so he could get better." I was dumbfounded. Could it really be that this valiant little boy had invited illness into his body, as a way to help his brother? I was incredibly touched. We tapped: *I was scared for my little brother and got sick instead. He got well, but I stayed sick. I thought I was doing a good thing to make him better. I didn't know he would get well on his own. Then I stayed sick. I am a good boy. I promised to get ill because I love my little brother so much. I chose to get ill for my brother, but I don't have to do that anymore. Now I know my brother will get well on his own, and I can get well too. I release myself from that promise to be ill for him. I can now get better.*

The tapping brought some relief, but there was still something lingering in his eyes. So I had him look at his disease again. This time it was a pain in his left chest/heart. I asked if he felt guilty and he did. We tapped: *I feel guilty because I promised to get sick so my brother could get well. I am a good kid doing what I thought was best. I didn't know better, but now I am free to heal too.* He looked so relieved. Afterwards he only wanted to close his eyes and sleep.

The next time I saw him he looked wonderful, happy and healthy. His father said he was doing well.

When I receive donations from the TappyBear Foundation (see Resources Section in back of book) I give TappyBears to the children. Emigdio now has his own TappyBear to use when at home. The smile on his face when he received his TappyBear was positively heart-melting. I *know* his life has changed for the better.

Jhenifher

I met Jhenifher the first day she arrived at the hospital, right after her diagnosis of leukemia. That very day I introduced her to TappyBear and EFT and showed her how to use her magic fingers. She tapped along with me on Tappy. We started with simple statements like: *I am a good girl; I am smart and lovely.* We tapped on her fear of being in the hospital, being ill and not getting better. As we tapped, we put all her fears in a red balloon and sent them away. She was all smiles.

Then next time I spoke to her she told me that she had been tapping and how good it made her feel. We tapped about her illness. She told me it was ugly. We tapped: *It is ugly. It is so ugly. It scares me. I don't understand it. I'm afraid of it. I can change it from ugly to something nice. I see it changing now. Now it is nice. I feel better.* We tapped about her body healing, and about feeling happy, good and healthy. We tapped: *I am valuable. I didn't do anything wrong even though my parents left me with my grandmother. I have lots of value just because I am me.*

I saw her three weeks later. She looked absolutely radiant and told me she felt good. She didn't have any pain, or fear. She had been tapping at home. I gave her a TappyBear and after that she tapped with him every day.

One day she was in for treatments and was told her blood sugar was too high. Two days before, she'd had visitors from her school (the whole class) who had brought her cake. Even though she had only eaten a small piece, her blood sugar had risen and she'd gotten dizzy. We tapped: *It is okay to have a piece of cake. It is okay to have visitors and be treated special. I am sweet. It is okay to be appreciated and supported. It is okay to receive. It is okay to have normal blood sugar.* The look on her face told me everything. She was not accustomed to having so many people be "sweet" to her. It had been too much, but now she knew she could receive that attention and not get out of balance.

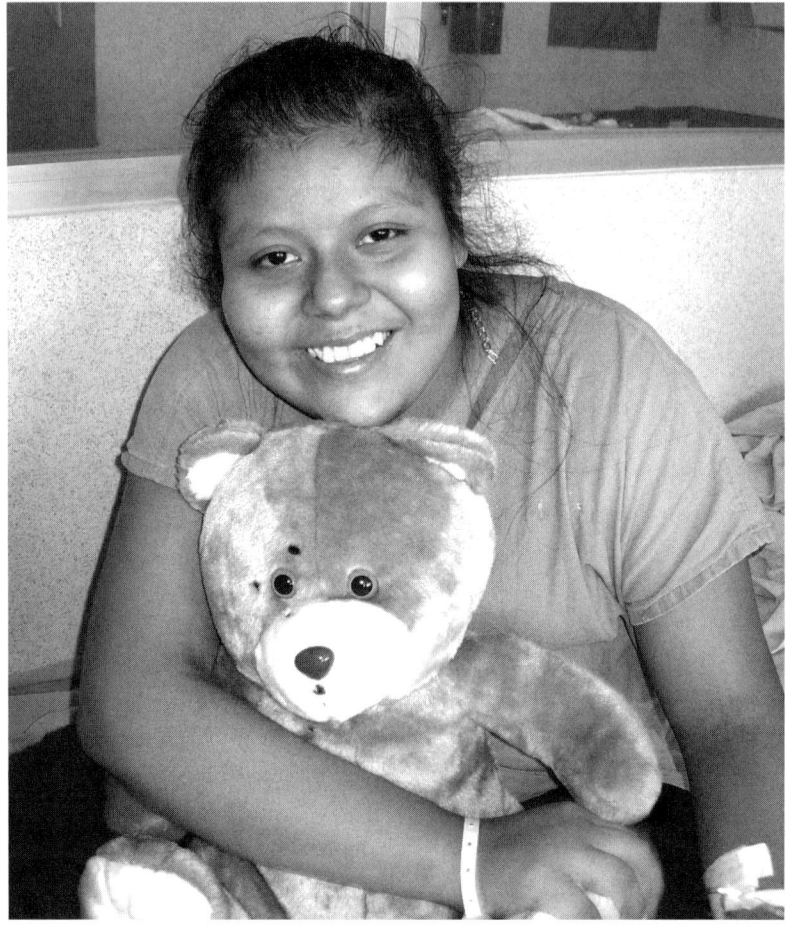

Jhenifher with Tappy.

One day her stomach hurt after she was given her meds. We tapped and imagined pink light there to protect her stomach from the medicines. She looked up and said the pain was gone. Then we chose an animal to represent her as "healthy." For Jhenifher it was, of course, a little bear. She told me she chose a bear because it is tender, smart, loving and gives lots of hugs. Then *I* got a hug from Jhenifher.

Jhenifher, like most of the other children on the ward, had to periodically receive an injection in the spinal column. Even though an analgesic is put on their back, they suffer from the shot. I saw Jhenifher after the injection and she told me that it really didn't hurt. I learned that she had told the doctor that since she'd been tapping with TappyBear, she didn't feel any pain.

As I got to know Jhenifher a little better, I found out that her father had left her brother and her when she was four years old. She didn't know why then and still doesn't. She has been living with her grandparents since then. We tapped: *Even though my father abandoned me, I'm a good girl. I am lovable. I didn't do anything wrong. I don't know what happened between my mother and father. They never told me but I am still a wonderful girl. It was not about me. It was an adult thing. I am valuable.* Then she told me she is afraid her grandfather will die. We tapped: *I'm afraid Grandpa will die and leave me. He will leave me just like my dad did. I wouldn't know how to find him. My dad calls me once in awhile, but how would I talk to Grandpa after he dies. I don't want to lose him too.* The fear of him dying was black. We tapped about this too. Her fear disappeared and she wasn't worried about him dying anymore. She wasn't worried about being abandoned.

Jhenifher is an excellent case because she taps and talks to her TappyBear all the time. She is motivated to tap, to feel good and to heal. She told me the other day that she is *certain* she will heal. You can't ask for any more than that from a sick child. That kind of confidence is pure gold.

Jhenifher asked me to be her godmother at her 15th birthday party. She is currently 11 years old. Why do I mention this? Because it shows she is planning for the future, not afraid of today or tomorrow. Most kids with leukemia have an intense fear of making any plans. Jhenifher is planning four years out into the future. She is definitely moving past all fears of illness because she is focusing what she desires for the future.

"I use TappyBear every day, all day, and I feel content," says Jhenifher. "I use Tappy to get rid of my fears especially when I have to come to the hospital. I feel so proud to have received Tappy. I want to go back to school so I can share my appreciation with my classmates and show them how to use Tappy to feel good too."

Rodolfo

Rodolfo is an 11-year-old boy who was back in the hospital because of pain in his stomach and side. He was diagnosed with a calcified mass in his right kidney. I tapped with him to get rid of that initial pain and from there on he began tapping with TappyBear as a daily ritual. I left a TappyBear with him in the hospital; he slept with it and tapped with it daily. Even when he went home he tapped every day. He promised to tap twice a day and he did. The results have been marvelous.

Rodolfo was scheduled for surgery to remove the kidney mass. He was afraid of this surgery and we tapped away all of those fears. Then we worked on the mass itself. We started by visualizing it. It was about the size of a grapefruit. We saw his precancerous cells encapsulated in light, just as a grapefruit has a skin around it.

I told Rodolfo to imagine doing whatever he needed to do to remove that mass and then asked him what that might be. He said, "Cut it out with a sword." We tapped: *I use my sword to cut that mass into pieces. I burn those bad cells until there is only ash left and I blow away the ashes. I change those bad cells into good cells. Even if the doctors need to take them out it is okay.* Once we did this he was no longer afraid of the surgery.

57

We continued: *I release any hidden fears and any need to cover them up so that I appear strong.* He began to yawn profusely as we tapped. (Yawning is a sign of release when tapping.) *I am a good boy, not a bad boy. I change my fears to strengths.*

We imagined how the surgery would go from beginning to end and tapped while we did it: *I am smiling and laughing with the nurses and doctors. They treat me really well. They take care of me. I go to sleep without worries. I know the surgeon is doing his best work. I take five angels with me to take care of me and the doctors and nurses. I come back to my room afterwards and feel fine.* He liked these images very much. He promised me that if he felt any fear when he was about to go to surgery he would tap.

In the end, the surgery was put off. This was his opportunity to tap to remove that mass!

Rodolfo promised to tap twice a day when at home (even without a TappyBear). He looked fabulous when I saw him again. He had great color, was smiling ear to ear and looked so very happy, even though he was waiting to have his appointment with the doctor. His stomach aches had gone away. He hadn't had a cold, which he usually got often.

I received some donations of TappyBears from the TappyBear Foundation (see Resources Section) and Rodolfo was one of the children who was given one. He beamed as he received his Tappy. He has been tapping with it every day since.

About three months after tapping (and receiving his chemotherapy), the doctor told Rodolfo that his tumor was *gone*. He is ecstatic. He will be returning to the hospital for checkups and precautionary treatments. He promised to keep tapping.

"Now that your tumor is gone," I told him, "I'd like to you tap on staying healthy and that tumor never coming back." We tapped: *I'm so happy that my tumor went away. I'm so glad it is gone. I want it to never come back again. I continue to tap that my body stays healthy, that I am nice to myself. I choose to be healthy until I'm 90 years old.*

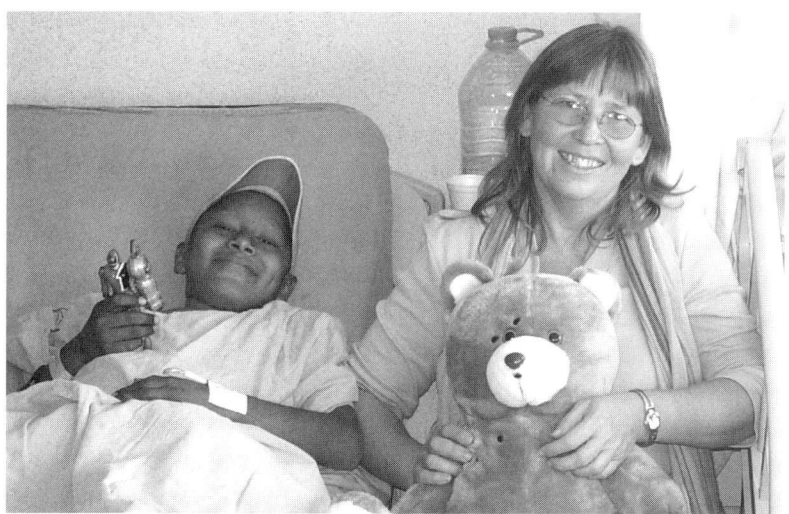

Rudolfo, Deborah, and Tappy.

The biggest grin broke out on his face as I mentioned being a healthy 90 years old. Obviously he had never thought about getting healthy, staying healthy and choosing to grow to be a healthy old man. He liked that a lot!

If children facing the fears and pains of something as terrifying as cancer can derive such great benefits from tapping with TappyBear, just imagine what Tappy can do for your child's "normal" aches, pains and fevers! It is worth trying on "everything" that may upset a child.

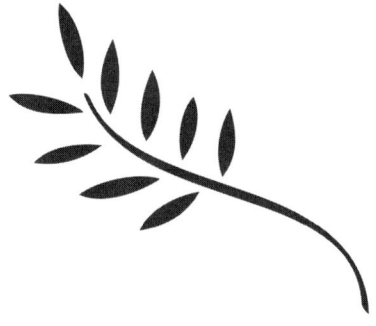

Chapter 5

How to Introduce Tappy to the Children in Your Life

One of the most beneficial things you can do when introducing TappyBear to a child is to first deal with any doubts or insecurities *you* may have about EFT. Is it going to work for this child? Will she *want* to tap on the EFT spots? Will an older child or teen think it's "silly" to tap on a toy bear or to repeat those words? Many questions may arise.

By far the best way to gain confidence about EFT *in general* is by learning it yourself. If you are not already an experienced "EFTer," you will probably want to discover its amazing benefits for yourself before using it on a child. Once you have been able to vanquish a toothache or improve your confidence at public speaking by the simple application of this short and painless technique, you will become a "believer." And "believers" make the best teachers, especially of children, who maybe filled with doubts and questions.

The important thing to remember is that if *you* are confident about the value of what you are doing and can understand the soothing effects of TappyBear, then you will easily convey this to a child. Children model themselves after older children or adults, especially their parents. They

61

will quickly absorb and reflect your own attitude about the bear. If you are dismissive or noncommittal, the child will likely be too. By tapping on and clearing your own beliefs first, you will be helping create powerful new beliefs for yourself and the children. That is why a bit of preparation on your part before introducing Tappy can go a long way toward making things go smoothly.

Till Schilling, Tappy's inventor, says that he almost always introduces Tappy by having the parent or adult receive him first. The child then wants to imitate the parent and eagerly presses for her own opportunity to use Tappy. Till's approach is to introduce the child to tapping slowly and in small doses, preserving the sense that Tappy is a special helper, not to be taken on too lightly or casually. This "reverence" and slow caution gives the child an ongoing appreciation for the true power of EFT, which shouldn't be treated offhandedly.

Deborah Miller, whose work with children in the cancer unit we read about earlier, points out that she has often seen the process work the reverse way as well. That is, the child falls in love with TappyBear and starts tapping with him first. The parents then see the value the child is getting from the experience, become interested and end up trying themselves.

For most of us, though, we'll be the ones to get the ball rolling and set the proper tone with Tappy and the child.

Handling Your Concerns about Using TappyBear with a Child

Here are some ways you can prepare yourself to present Tappy effectively and with confidence. Do this *before* introducing Tappy to the child.

1) "Tap" on yourself using an EFT phrase like:

Even though I have fears about introducing TappyBear and EFT to this child, I choose to fully and deeply believe that it will help..

Even though I'm worried about how to introduce TappyBear to this child, I choose to experience the fun of TappyBear and convey that feeling.

Even though I don't know what to say when I introduce TappyBear, I choose to look right into Tappy's eyes and let "him" dictate the words to say.

Even though I'm uncertain about how to introduce TappyBear I choose to feel fully confident and show my own enjoyment of Tappy as I talk

With a teenager, for instance, you might be afraid that they will mock you or think you've "gone nuts." Your fear may stem from thinking that they are too old for teddy bears, and that tapping is really weird to begin with. As much as we may hate to admit it, we want to feel accepted and respected by our children (especially our teenagers). In part, you may also fear that your child's possible doubts and protests will overcome your confidence. Or you might feel that you don't want to make things worse by "pushing" something new onto an already problematic situation.

Tap on all of these types of concerns. Keep tapping until you feel you've uncovered and addressed all of your own hidden attitudes and issues. It's important to remember that you do this as much for yourself as for the child. The child will benefit from tapping, often in spite of your attitude, but when you "clean up" your own attitude, you will be much more likely to *encourage* a child to tap as a first defense when she's hurting and to support her in making EFT a "normal" part of her life.

2) Become more informed about EFT

Refresh yourself about the extraordinary benefits other adults and children have received from EFT by reading articles and testimonials on the websites listed in the Resources Section or in books you can borrow or buy, or that you may already own. An excellent overall introduction to EFT, its benefits and uses, is Dr. Carrington's book, *Try It On Everything: Discover the Power of EFT* (see Resources section for details).

Remember why you ordered this special bear in the first place. You probably ordered it through a recommendation of someone you trust or after seeing or reading about the benefits another child gained from using Tappy. The more you discover about what it has done for others, the more creative and optimistic you will be about the benefits your own child may receive.

Simply put, he more you know about EFT, the better a coach and guide you will be. Fortunately, EFT is an elegantly simple tool, so it doesn't take long to become an "expert." Just do some reading and, if possible, talk to others who have successfully used it.

3) Trust in EFT, Tappy and your Child

You have already read in Chapter 3 some awe-inspiring stories about what EFT, and Tappy, has done for children. The possibilities are vast, and, with your own creativity and intuition, you will find new ways to bring Tappy into the life of a child. Trust that your child is going to receive great benefit, and approach the whole exchange with that attitude in your heart. To give you a good start, I have outlined some suggestions just in case you need them.

"Tappy is Your Special Friend"

In general, it is extremely beneficial to introduce Tappy as the child's buddy (choose the appropriate word —

friend, pal, helper, confidant, etc.— depending on the age and personality of the child). This works with every age, including adults. Tappy's special features — his gentle eyes, perked ears, size and "snuggle factor"— make him irresistible. Even the most hardened, "world-damaged" soul warms to him, though they may not always show it. This is especially true if he is given as a gift to the child, but it works just as well in a therapeutic setting.

When the child visits for therapy, make sure they know that Tappy is there for them — that Tappy wants to sit with them or "hang out" with them during the session.

Even if the child never taps with Tappy, it is important to remember that Tappy is still doing some good. For to have such an accepting and open friend is a need of everyone. Even without tapping, the child will feel the acceptance and compassion that Tappy offers, and this is often all that they need. To be able to hug Tappy, cry with him, look into his eyes and even get angry at him when the child is upset is a great gift.

Good Friends are Listeners

When introducing Tappy, you might tell the child that a best friend is a *listening* friend and that Tappy is there to listen to anything that they need to say about anything at all. Children of all ages (and, again, adults too) can feel free to express deep emotions and uncover sensitive memories when they know that: (1) they are being heard, (2) the listener will not judge them or think less of them, and (3) the listener will keep their secret safe.

When children *express* their suffering — even when no one but Tappy hears — it *releases* that pain. In time, the pain lessens to the point at which the child may be able to talk about it with their parents or therapist. Ultimately, though, it is *hearing their own voice* speak those feelings that has the power to heal. And Tappy serves as a marvelous "sounding board" for this purpose.

Tappy Needs Your Help

As we saw in Dr. Immergluck's article, Tappy can be introduced to children as someone a bit like themselves, someone who has the same pain or problem they have. For instance, if a child has trouble sleeping, you might say, *Tappy is really tired and he can't go to sleep. Maybe you can help him?* Children will often respond with compassion to this. After all, the child knows what this problem feels like. They will be more likely to help someone (Tappy) in need when they *understand* this need. In their efforts to help Tappy overcome the same issue, the child learns how to help himself as well.

This type of introduction will more likely be successful with younger children — generally ages 0 to 7. During these years, children are more likely to consider a stuffed animal or doll to be "real"— a living being with feelings. It's important to know the child in order to decide whether or not this would be the best approach. Remember, though, that any approach you take cannot be a "mistake." All of us need to help others, whether we show it or not. And when we are given the space to do this, even for a stuffed bear, it changes us.

Be Prepared to Talk About the Tapping Spots

A child will typically ask, right away, the purpose of the buttons on Tappy. Knowing just a bit about EFT can go a long way toward providing a satisfying answer. When the child asks about the buttons, as she inevitably will, here's an example of what you might say:

The buttons on Tappy's fur have a special purpose. They are placed on certain spots on his body that, when tapped very gently, make him feel better about what is making him upset. When you tap on the buttons, one by one, and speak a sentence about how he feels, it can make his sadness go away. When you tap the buttons, you might say: "Even though I miss my Mommy, I am a great bear!" Would you like to try to help him feel better about being away from his Mommy? It's fun, and Tappy will feel much better.

The child may also ask about the correct order of the buttons. You can show her the usual order that is used in tapping, but also tell her if she taps "incorrectly," it's okay. The main purpose is to allow children to speak their own pain as they are healing Tappy, vicariously, of their own suffering.

Using first person "I" as the child taps on TappyBear is extremely beneficial because the mind hears this sentence repeated again and again... even though the child is not a "bear." The child, in the above example, misses her mother, and tapping the phrase, *Even though I miss my Mommy, I am a great bear,* works so well, the last word makes no real difference.

68

Tappy is a Helper Bear, and He Can Teach You How to Heal Yourself

One of Tappy's most helpful qualities is that the exact EFT spots are represented on his fur in a way that anyone can understand. It can be hard for a child to learn how to tap on his or her own body. Being "taught" by an adult means being touched and, for many reasons, it is not always appropriate for an adult friend, relative, social worker, teacher or counselor to touch the child. Sometimes, due to circumstances that might very well be related to the child's pain, it is not even appropriate for the *parent* to touch the child in order to show them the EFT spots. With TappyBear, however, children can practice the EFT spots on Tappy while learning to tap those spots on their own bodies.

Use the TappyBear Songs to Introduce Him

Special Tappy songs on a CD and on the TappyBear website are available. Having the child listen to them and Tap Along With Tappy is an easy and enjoyable way to introduce the concept of tapping away one's troubles with EFT. (See www.tappybear.com for more information).

Trust Your Intuition and Your Knowledge of the Child

Depending on the age of the child, one or more of the above suggestions might be helpful. However, as always, your intuition is the key, and only you know what the child in your life needs.

One way you might look at introducing Tappy is as a progression:

1) You present the child with a good friend.

2) You build a sense of trust in the child by letting them know that Tappy will listen to them.

3) You build a sense of compassion and service by helping the child understand that Tappy needs help and shares their same pain.

4) You show the child how to help Tappy through EFT.

5) You help the child *understand* how Tappy is helping them through EFT.

Through this progression, or the progression you feel makes the most sense for your particular child, there are very few kids or adults who will not, in time, respond to TappyBear. Some children respond very quickly and "adopt" Tappy right out of the box. Others take longer. Be patient. Tappy works and EFT works. Even the smallest of us recognize healing when it happens, and children warm quickly the idea of healing themselves and others. The key is to stick with it, as Till Schilling did with Christine in Chapter 3.

Healing the suffering of children is perhaps the most vital and valuable act we can perform as stewards of our planet. Introducing kids to TappyBear, though sometimes difficult, is a great gift to them. If we remember this, even the most difficult moments become moments of strength-building and precious lessons to learn.

A child who grows up using TappyBear and EFT will likely grow into an adult who generously spreads healing energy in the world.

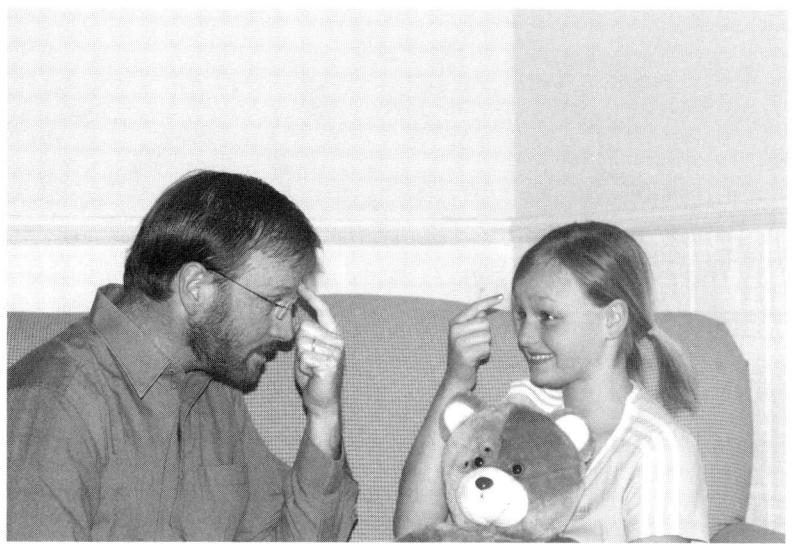

Tapping with Tappy brings family members together.

Chapter 6

TappyBear for Adults

Looking back over this guide, I ask you — what grownup would not be deeply comforted by being able to use their own TappyBear?

Wouldn't it be wonderful if a good friend were to say to you: *Open this box I wrapped for you. This friendly bear is yours. He's a good friend, a good hugger, an open listener, and he accepts everything about you. You can talk to him when you are too ashamed to speak to anyone else. You can heal him when he suffers like you do. He is yours.*

Would you not be overjoyed? Would you, too, not find him of great help?

Many times, I have found TappyBear to be amazingly valuable to me when nothing else seemed to comfort me during difficult times. In the following article that I wrote for my newsletter, *EFT 1-Minute News,* you can see how transferring my stress and fear onto Tappy made all the difference.

How "TappyBear" Helped to Handle a Troublesome Situation

Recently I had an experience that opened up for me

a new understanding of what Gary Craig, founder of EFT, calls "tail enders"— those nagging inner doubts and contradictions that beset us as we try to face a problem rationally. They are the "yes, buts…" which can be created by our minds in almost every situation. These are the single greatest obstacle to having EFT (or any treatment for that matter) work successfully.

There is not a single person who has ever used EFT who has not run into the problem of tail enders and had to address it sooner or later.

I'd like to give you a little background on what happened to me the other night when I myself used TappyBear, so you will understand what my anxiety and frustration was about. If you are not an experienced computer user you may want to skip the following few paragraphs and just sum it all up in your mind as "Pat Carrington's despair at seeming to lose nine years of critical data on her computer" and let it go at that. If you're curious to hear the actual story, read on!

After acting up badly for two weeks, my computer ended up in the computer repair store and was ultimately unable to be repaired. Dell sent out a repair person to the store because my computer was still on warranty, but that unfortunately made it worse. The company had already replaced two motherboards and three audio cards since I bought it two years ago. Now they had to wipe the disk. So I dutifully backed up all my data onto an external hard drive and comforted myself with the knowledge that I would also have my daily internet-driven backups to rely on for safety. Little did I know… most of my back-up efforts turned out to be futile.

When I purchased a new computer — the old one was of no use now except perhaps as an emergency backup – and went to restore the data from my external hard drive, neither my new computer nor any of my friends' computers could recognize the external hard drive. When I took the drive to the computer repair people they tested it and said, "We can't imagine why, but that drive is fried!" Which meant, quite simply, that everything on it was recoverable only if I paid thousands of dollars to a recovery center to reconstruct the data.

Since Dell had wiped the old computer, and the external drive was unusable, I began to run a "restore" on my online backup service, which would mean I would only lose two weeks of data from the time my old computer had been disabled. Since the restore was going to take a long time, I went to sleep easily.

Waking in the middle of the night I decided to find out what had happened with the restore. I clicked to extract the file that presumably had been downloaded. It had indeed been downloaded, but the extracting system was unable to make my files available! It said my files could not be opened. Suddenly, though I had held up through all the various stages of this problem so far, there set in a sense of "catastrophe." What seemed to me to be my last hope for recovering my data was now telling me it was unrecoverable!

I at least had enough sense to use EFT for this.

After a couple of rounds of EFT, using the EFT statement, "Even though I have no access to my stored data, I choose to handle this situation calmly and effectively," I felt a bit better but was still burningly aware of the fact that essential data containing hundreds of valuable contacts, unduplicated writings which I had always intended to get back to, earlier versions of many projects, and an incredible amount of valuable information about EFT that people had sent to me over the years, was in jeopardy. I had chosen to be optimistic and creative in my approach but it looked at that moment to be a total disaster.

The tapping did make some difference, of course, but it was slow going because of a compelling voice in the back of my head telling me over and over again that I was facing an insurmountable obstacle.

Then I got an idea. Sitting across the room from me, seated comfortably on my stationary reclining bicycle, was my EFT Bear, "Tappy." This soft and friendly creature is always a reminder to me of much wisdom that I can sometimes forget. I need only look into his earnest face to feel different about any issue at hand. I say this with emphasis because I see him as quite unlike ordinary teddy bears with their widely spaced button-like eyes that do not look directly at one, and their flat faces and inconspicuous ears. *Tappy's* eyes are set in the front of his face exactly as are human eyes, so he seems to look right into your own eyes, to be "real" in a sense. I can only describe the expression on this toy bear's face, as I looked at him at that moment, as one of concern and attention. There was nothing superficial about his appearance. His ears faced forward alertly so that they seemed to listen to every word that I was repeating as I held him. Interestingly enough, this experience using Tappy has given me an entirely new slant on the "tail ender" problem.

75

There are many ways that any of us can use TappyBear. Both children and adults can complain to Tappy about things they cannot easily tell others. The sincere face of the listening bear seems to absorb their complaints with no judgment whatsoever, so that as they tap they become quieter and quieter — the familiar response of many children to EFT.

This soft and gentle bear is an ever-present ambassador of EFT, extending its help to us under many different conditions. This particular night, truly upset by the computer problem, I first had to decide just how to use this assistance. Would I simply complain to him out loud while tapping on him, or me? Or should I surrogate-tap on him, holding the bear, pretending that he had lost his computer data and attempting to help him out of his despair and anger?

I decided on the latter course because I like to extend help, which is probably why I am a therapist. It almost invariably does wonderful things for me. So I decided to pretend that the bear had experienced the same computer disaster I had and I would try to help him.

I started by tapping on the soft fuzzy side of his paw and repeating the phrase, "Even though Tappy has no access to his precious data, I choose to have him be optimistic and creative in how he handles this."

When I had said this three times while tapping on the Karate Chop spot, his sad expression seemed to change and he looked almost like a different bear. This was a perfect example of how projecting our own feelings into an external object (person, animal or toy) seems to change that object before our very eyes as we tap. We often, in fact, understand our own dilemmas more clearly when we are dealing with someone other than ourselves, because by so doing we are bypassing the "tail enders" that are built into us.

When I tapped on all the EFT spots on the bear, doing an abbreviated version of the *EFT Choices Method*, it worked immediately. After only one round of tapping, during which I felt increasing sympathy for this little fellow, I saw something of great interest when I looked into his earnest face. A thought occurred to me that might well have come to me after several rounds of ordinary EFT, but would have been unlikely to have happened so quickly.

I saw *Tappy* differently. I now saw him as undergoing something that would actually help him grow up to be a more resourceful little person/bear. Just as a parent does not want their child to face certain hardships but knows that this is going to strengthen the child, I felt this with *Tappy*. In fact I could feel it more easily for Tappy than I could have for myself. In effect, Tappy was acting as my surrogate and thereby helping me to bypass the conditionings that can make us unable to access solutions and get out of ourselves.

I could see my own dilemma "from the outside" as I held him. As I experienced his softness and innocence, as I patted his head and held him, I found myself changing the EFT Statement the second time around to add the words "right now" to the end of the negative statement, so it now went, "Even though Tappy has no access to his precious data *right now*...". When we tapped on this I seemed to see the little fellow appraising the whole situation differently and recognizing that while *right now* he had no access to the data, this might be reversed tomorrow when proper technical help was available.

I now took my own Distress Level (SUDS level), which had been an 8 before we started EFT. It had come down to about a 2 and Tappy now "looked" to me as though he realized ("he" being me of course!) that the world hadn't come to an end because of what was happening.

I next noticed that "he" seemed tired and angry at the series of continual frustrations that this whole situation had imposed upon him! This was a new Aspect. So we started tapping on "his" feeling of anger. It was pretty strong — a 4 to a 6. As I tapped on him, I was saying, "Even though Tappy is angry because he has all these obstacles to deal with, I choose to have him triumph and become stronger because of them."

He seemed to watch me seriously, his lovely round eyes fixated upon my face, as I repeated the EFT phrases that I hoped could help him become stronger and triumph over this difficulty. As I did so, a whole philosophy of life seemed to emerge. As the little bear sat there patiently, he seemed to represent all of us when we wish things would go differently for ourselves and those we love. As I tapped, an inner voice seemed to be saying, "When you get stronger and better and more competent, you're more happy about yourself."

I ended up feeling peaceful, went quietly to sleep, and awoke in the morning with many solutions in my mind. I was eventually able to overcome the difficulties involved in getting the special tech support I needed. There were several more obstacles to surmount, of course, but my feeling about them was entirely different. I had bypassed my tail enders, thanks to a meaningful session with a golden bear named Tappy.

Advantages to Using Tappy as an Adult

EFT, as you know by now, is a wonderful, self-administered technique that "resets" the energy system as we tap on our acupressure points. Since adults can use EFT anytime and anyplace, *without* the benefit of a stuffed toy, why might they *want* to use TappyBear? What advantages might TappyBear give us over tapping, bear-free? Here are just a few...

Tappy Serves as a Great Reminder

Oddly enough, one of the greatest practical drawbacks to EFT is simply that people forget to use it! Often I listen to people who have used EFT successfully — even "miraculously" — in the past, as they describe some present struggle they are going through. The first question I usually ask is, "Have you tried EFT on it?" I can't tell you how often I am met by a prolonged silence, followed by a, "Hmm, I didn't think of that. I really should try it, I guess."

I think many people still secretly believe EFT is "too good to be true," even after they have repeatedly used it successfully. So they don't consider it a first line of defense. Or they forget the pain they were in before using EFT, so they minimize the importance of the technique. Or they convince themselves that the reason their problem cleared up was something other than EFT. Whatever the reason, many of us often simply forget to use EFT when a new problem arises in their lives.

Simply by having a TappyBear on display in a prominent place in our homes, we are constantly reminded of the healing power of this astonishing technique. Tappy silently implores us to tap when we're in pain or struggle, or when we want to make positive change in some area of our lives. That alone makes him worth having, even if we never lay a hand on him. He keeps the presence of EFT alive in our minds.

Tappy Sparks Insight

One of the best ways to come up with powerful tapping statements and uncover hidden aspects of our fears is by helping — or *pretending* to help — someone else who shares the same problem we have. Many of us think more clearly about a problem and see more obvious solutions when it is another person we are helping, not ourselves.

By pretending Tappy has the very issue we are working on, we free ourselves up to think more objectively and creatively about the problem. My computer story is one example of this. We also saw Tappy used in this way with a child's anxieties in an earlier story.

It may feel strange at first to play helper to TappyBear, but the awkwardness quickly disappears as we see the power of this method. By helping Tappy, we "step out of" our own problem and are able to look at it at a greater distance, and with more compassion and clarity.

Tappy Is a Non-Judgmental "Partner"

Sometimes we tap about "embarrassing" or deeply personal issues we are not comfortable sharing with others. Yet, at the same time, we wish we could have some help and support. TappyBear makes an excellent companion and helper in these instances. He plays the open, friendly and utterly non-judgmental partner as we open up about our most guarded thoughts and feelings.

Tappy never judges or condemns. He never rejects us or withdraws. He is just *there* to help us voice our most intimate struggles and to provide warm support. Using Tappy to help us resolve sensitive issues is one of his mot powerful contributions.

Tappy "Speaks" to the Child in Us

On some level, none of us ever really grow up. Yes, we acquire new experiences and perspectives, but the child within us remains essentially unchanged. Unfortunately, many of us learn to bury and ignore that child as we immerse ourselves more and more in the world of adult worries and concerns.

TappyBear is a wonderful, natural way for us to honor and care for the child within us. By making contact with the innocent, vulnerable inner child, we move ourselves closer to the place where genuine healing occurs.

Tappy is a helper for all ages…

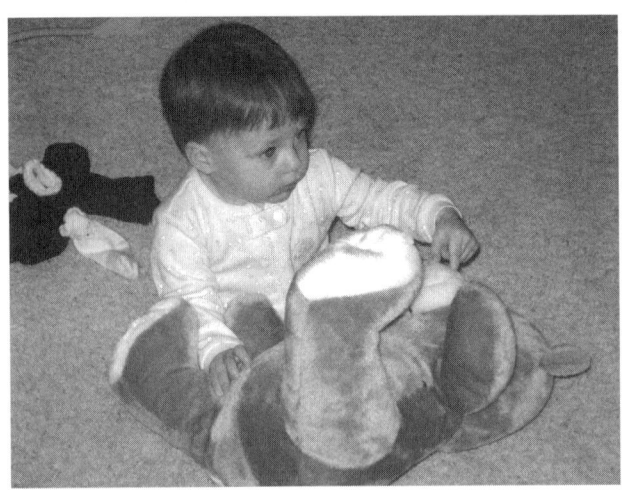

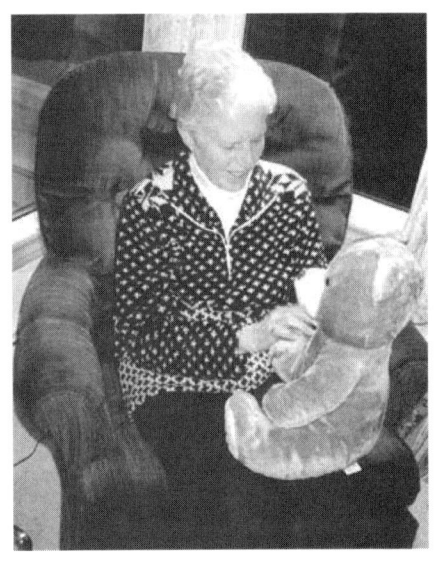

Tappy Give Us a Chance to "Spread the Word" About EFT

TappyBear is a terrific conversation starter with both grownups and children. When we carry him about or prop him up in a special place in our home, office or dorm room, he invites others to ask us about him (after all, he's not your "average bear"). This gives us a wonderful opportunity to talk about EFT to friends, colleagues and family members.

Many of us who have tried EFT naturally want to "share the wealth" with people we love and care about. But we are reluctant to appear to be proselytizing. TappyBear creates an open invitation for others to ask us about him and, by association, EFT. It is always easier and more effective to share information about a helping technique when someone *asks* us about it than when we bombard them with, "I know a great new technique you should try." When we share from the latter posture, people immediately put up their defenses, but when they *ask* us, their minds are open to receive.

Tappy "Teaches" EFT

Whether we're learning EFT for the first time, re-learning it after setting it aside for a while, or teaching it to a child or fellow grownup, Tappy stands as a beautiful, silent guide to the tapping points. Simply by looking at Tappy, we know where to tap on ourselves. By allowing Tappy to serve as a visual guide, we lower the anxiety for others who are learning EFT for the first time. They don't need to keep asking us where the tapping points are, or worry that they're getting it wrong, they need only glance at Tappy.

So if you're in any kind of healing or counseling position in which you sometimes teach EFT, having a TappyBear on hand is a great learning aid.

I'm sure you'll come up with your own "adult" reasons for inviting TappyBear into your home!

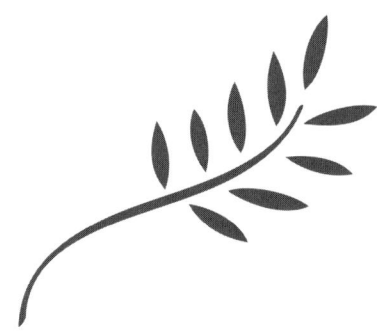

Chapter 7
Concluding Thoughts

It seems odd to attribute healing qualities to a stuffed bear, but once you have worked with TappyBear yourself and seen him "do his thing" with children, I think you'll agree that Tappy seems to possess an almost magical ability to advance the healing power of EFT.

Of course, TappyBear doesn't possess any actual power of his own. As I have suggested many times in this small book, Tappy's real magic is in the way he reflects and reveals the power we all have within us. Tappy possesses only the healing properties that we give him, but those properties can often take us by surprise when they seem to "pour" directly from a warm and cuddly stuffed bear's eyes. Tappy can help anyone, from the most innocent child to the grumpiest grownup, unlock the powers of EFT in ways we can't always do on our own.

However, Tappy is not required in order for EFT to work. EFT is a remarkable technique that is designed to work completely on its own, using only our fingers and our words. It has been employed by thousands of people around the world to ease pain, dissolve phobias, cure allergies, improve performance, aid weight loss, neutralize painful memories, and help with dozens of other issues.

Its strength lies in its ability to cut directly to the *source* of pain — those disrupted energy signals in our bodies.

But Tappy certainly brings a new *dimension* to EFT. He offers children a lovable, huggable companion who will not only "hold their hands" as they tap through their fears and pains, but can also — often without the child consciously realizing it — serve as an emotional "stand-in" for the child him — or herself. As the child helps Tappy with "his problems," or offers Tappy as an aid to other children, this child is unleashing his or her own healing powers and insights. What the child does for and with Tappy, she is really doing for and with herself. It's really quite extraordinary.

TappyBear offers a whole new way to make the remarkable powers of EFT accessible to children. He helps take EFT out of the realm of "weird adult behavior" and make it simple, immediate, useful — and fun! — for children. At the same time, Tappy provides an extremely effective healing tool for adults. After all, many of the pains and fears for which we *use* EFT actually started in childhood. How wonderful to have this wise-but-innocent stuffed companion who can lead us back to the forgotten realm of the child within, that child who may have been hurt so very long ago and just needs to be touched and loved in order to heal. *We* may have forgotten this inner child, but Tappy hasn't. Tappy knows how to make instant contact.

There are countless ways to use TappyBear for our children and ourselves, but ultimately, the best way is the way that *you* will use him. You may come up with approaches no one has ever tried before. Feel free to experiment. Tappy will never hurt you or steer you astray. You can't "do it wrong." And if you should discover some fabulous new way to unleash his (your) inner powers, please write and tell us all about it. We love collecting Tappy stories. And who knows — your story might be just the inspiration some despairing parent needs to try the life-changing powers of EFT on a hurting child. And that act may change countless lives.

Tappy, I honestly believe, is a force for good in this world. And therefore I recommend that you always treat him with respect. He will return the favor tenfold, believe me. Handle him gently. Speak to him softly. When you're done using him, "tuck him away" in a special place; don't just toss him on the floor. After all, you wouldn't want to be treated that way! And what we do to Tappy we do to ourselves.

So do me a favor, will you? Pick up Tappy right now and give him a great big, mushy hug. Know that this is my way of hugging *you* and thanking you for helping to spread the "miracle of EFT" to another child or grownup. The world needs more healing. The world needs more compassion. The world needs more joy. EFT, along with its faithful champion, TappyBear, is an amazing way to bring a little more of all these good things into the world.

Happy tapping!!

Appendix A
Helpful Resources

Websites

Tappybear.com This site is the home of TappyBear and a major source of up-to-date information and helpful tips for adults and a delightful visiting spot for children in its "Kid's Corner". It is here that you can find up-to-date advice on the use of Tappy for many new issues, share your own stories and photos of TappyBear, and help your child learn about Tappy and EFT through downloading special coloring pages, listening to CDs with Tappy songs and stories on them, finding out where Tappy "lives" in the world, and engaging in other fun tasks. This lively, constantly updated site is a must for those who appreciate TappyBear. Go to **www.tappybear.com**.

MasteringEFT.com This inviting website is hosted by EFT Master **Dr. Patricia Carrington**. The site contains fascinating information on EFT, previews of Dr. Carrington's unique EFT training materials, and many special offers. It is a major site for those who wish to know more about EFT, why it works, how it can be expanded, what is new and exciting in this area. Go to **www.masteringeft.com**.

Emofree.com This important website is hosted by the Founder of EFT, Gary Craig. It's a major EFT resource containing literally thousands of reports by users from all parts of the world detailing various uses of EFT. It also sells Gary Craig's masterful collection of original EFT training materials and EFT Certification materials. Use its Search feature to find out just about anything you need to know about EFT's use and applications. Go to **www. emofree.com.**

SchoolMadeMuchEasier.com This valuable website is dedicated to everyone concerned with children's learning. It contains a wealth of useful resources for families and educators and very large active support community, making this site a must for anyone who wants to use EFT to enhance the learning experience. Host Paul Widdershoven has assembled a library of EFT guiding videos specifically for children, parents and teachers, as well as online seminars and webinars to support an ever growing community of school teachers and councilors who embrace EFT as their favorite "helping tool" for children. Go to **www.SchoolMadeMuchEasier.com.**

Newsletters

The Tappy Times This entertaining and instructive newsletter keeps parents and children up to date with the antics of TappyBear and motivates children to use EFT for many varying children's issues. Its up-to-date features makes it a lively source of information and special resources. To subscribe, go to **www.Tappybear.com.**

EFT 1-Minute News This major newsletter supplies you with a brief, lively, twice monthly report about what is going on in the world of EFT and the newest innovations that you can use to enrich EFT practice. Edited by EFT Master Dr. Patricia Carrington, it is widely recognized as a valuable source of in-depth information about EFT. When you subscribe to this free newsletter, you receive a bonus e-book by Dr. Carrington. To subscribe, go to **www.MasteringEFT.com**.

EFTInsights This newsletter, edited by the founder of EFT, Gary Craig, is the major source of reports from real life users of EFT. It is a must for serious students of EFT. To subscribe, go to **www.emofree.com.**

Publications

North Star Family Matters This heartwarming, highly readable family magazine which appears monthly is dedicated to inspiring conscious parenting and creating empowered kids. It consistently brings out the best in many of its avid subscribers as well as online visitors. The magazine is a favorite among well rounded parents who recognize the fact that we ourselves are children of an old way, yet the parents of a new consciousness. The editors are devoted users of both EFT and TappyBear. For information go to **www.familymatters.com.**

EFT Teaching Materials

First Steps in EFT (DVD) This short, simple, authoritative introduction to EFT for adults can't be beat for its convenience to new users of this method. EFT Master Dr. Patricia Carrington teaches all the basics of EFT in less than one hour, and provides all the training necessary to start a listener using EFT right away. As she leads you through "tapping" on an issue of your own, she also teaches you to apply the theory of Aspects and the Tearless Trauma technique to maximize the effects of EFT. To order go to **www.masteringeft.com.**

Try It On Everything: Discover the Power of EFT (Book) This comprehensive and enjoyable book gives you a complete and authoritative understanding of EFT — its origins, how and why it works, the scientific proof to date, and how to apply it to issues in your own life. It presents fascinating real life stories of people who have used it for countless problems of many different sorts and gives detailed accounts of the use of EFT by those whom we can see treated with this method in the movie by the same name (the companion film to this book, Try It On Everything). To order go to **www.masteringeft.com.**

Multiply the Power of EFT: 52 New Ways to Use EFT That Most People Don't Know About (Book) This book is for you if you already know EFT and want to greatly magnify its impact on your life. A veritable treasure trove of ideas and suggestions, this inspired volume will help you build EFT into a regular part of your life and use it to enhance your positive potential and self-esttem.

An invaluable resource for those who want to learn more about and get the most out of the technique. To order go to **www.masteringeft.com.**

How to Locate an EFT Therapist

When your problems or those of your child are deep seated in nature, it may well be wise to seek the assistance of an EFT Practitioner trained in the area of distress for which you wish help.

Because of the lack of centralization in EFT training, it is important that when you look for an EFT Practitioner you do so with as much information on hand as you can obtain. For this purpose, Dr. Carrington has written an important advisory e-Book entitled *A Guide to Finding an EFT Practitioner* which can be downloaded free of charge from her website **www.MasteringEFT.com.** If you are searching for a suitable EFT practitioner, we recommend that you first *print out and read this Guide.* It will help you evaluate the names you can obtain from the two major lists of EFT Practitioners: the list of EFT Certificate holders from the former EFT Certificate Program (see **www. masteringeft.com**) and Gary Craig's list of practitioners on his website (**www.emofree.com**). Neither of these lists are exhaustive and they partially overlap each other, but by using them you can readily locate practitioners in your vicinity for in-office treatment, or worldwide for telephone therapy, and then apply to them the evaluation criteria suggested by Dr. Carrington. In addition, the **www.tappybear.com** website has information about practitioners trained to treat children using TappyBear.

Appendix B

EFT Instructions

(NOTE: The following instructions represent a slight variation on Gary Craig's original Short Form sequence as published in his manual. I have added an additional tapping point, the Top of the Head Spot, to his sequence. Gary frequently uses this head spot when leading people through EFT and he finds it valuable, as do I and many others)

Instructions:

(1) Select the issue you want to work on and create in your mind a "scene", as from a movie, which typifies this issue for you. Thinking of that scene, select a "Distress Rating" (technically known as a SUDS rating) on a scale where "0" means that you are totally at ease about the situation depicted in the scene and have no problem with it at all, and a rating of "10" means that you are feeling as intensely (or distressed) as you possibly can imagine about this situation. The number that *first pops into your head* is your Distress Rating before commencing the technique — don't think too much about what the number should be and be sure to rate yourself on how you feel *right now,*

not how you expect to feel, or how you *did* feel.

(2) Create a key sentence (your Set-Up phrase) to use at the start of each "round" of the technique. The sentence goes like this:

> *Even though I am (feel, have, etc.)* _____ *(insert appropriate adjective describing your distress) at/ about, etc.* _____ *(insert name of person or situation involved), I deeply and completely accept myself.*

It makes no difference whether you *believe* that you deeply and profoundly accept yourself, just say it when the appropriate time comes.

When inserting the adjective that describes your feelings — make it a strong one. *Don't water down the feeling.* If you are furious or enraged or *deeply angry*, use those words and not more diplomatic, less intense words such as "annoyed" — later on, as your distress rating goes down, you will change the words you use in the sentence to match your feelings as they become less intense.

The reason for saying this sentence is that when we are caught in intense emotions, we tend to blame ourselves for having them. This sentence gets us "off our own back" and allows us to forgive ourselves for the feeling — this way the feeling can be dealt with much more easily.

Another thing to know about this method is that as your distress rating goes down (from "round" to "round") on the *first* emotion you address, other emotions that have been hidden beneath this one may surface — for example, underneath anger there may be a hidden fear, or grief, or other strong feelings. As these come up to the surface (as the first one lessens) they should be dealt with in turn. Use your intuition and change your sentence accordingly, giving yourself a new Severity Rating for this a *new* emotion, and do the tapping sequence to neutralize this feeling as well.

(3) Do this Preparation Exercise::

Locate the *Karate Chop Spot* (see photo below). It is on the outer, soft side of the hand, half way between

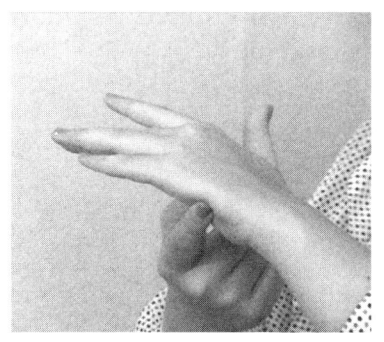

the base knuckle of the little finger and the wrist bone — this is the spot where the Karate "chop" is made when Karate masters split wood with their hand. You briskly tap this spot while saying the sentence you have created to yourself *out loud* 3 times.

(4) Do the Technique Proper.

Each time you move to a different spot in the sequence (see list below) you are to repeat an *abbreviated* form of your original sentence, called the Reminder Phrase It omits the phrases, "even though" and "deeply and profoundly accept myself" and leaves the rest of the sentence intact. For example, if your sentence had been "Even though I'm afraid of what might happen, I deeply and completely accept myself", then, as you moved from tapping-spot to tapping-spot, you would repeat to yourself a shorter version of this phrase such as "I'm afraid of what might happen." Or "I have this fear of what might happen", or even just, "this fear of what might happen". You say this

95

shorter sentence each time you move to a new tapping spot. Doing this keeps your mind focused on the problem that you are working on.

(5) Tap lightly but vigorously on each spot (as listed below) for as *many taps as it takes to complete your shorter sentence out loud* — then move to the next spot. It usually takes about 7 taps per spot to do this, but the exact number is unimportant.

The sequence of tapping points is as follows (see chart of face, upper body and hands). You can use either hand, and can tap on either side of the body:

Spot 1:   The Karate Chop Spot on side of hand.

Spot 2:   Inner corner of eyebrow.

Spot 3:   Outer corner of eye.

Spot 4:   Underneath the eye on the orbital bone, the bony structure beneath the eye (tap gently here, the tissue is delicate beneath the eyes).

Spot 5:   Directly beneath the nose (above the mouth).

Spot 6:   Directly beneath the mouth.

Spot 7:   Collarbone spot.   Make a fist and thump lightly on this spot, so that your fist covers the area just below one of the little points of the collarbone. Using your whole fist ensures that you are stimulating the entire area, it is therefore not necessary to be too precise with this location.

Spot 8: Underneath the arm at the side of upper chest, about 4 inches below the armpit (*exact position not essential*, see chart).

Spot 9. At the top of the head, near the front of the head. Curl your fingers downward so that the finger tips lightly tap the top of the head, positioning your hand with your wrist toward the front, your fingers pointing backwards, so that half of your fingers are stimulating the right side of your head and the remaining ones the left side — this stimulates both hemispheres of the brain. You may tap longer on this spot than the others if you wish.

This sequence completes one "round" of the treatment.

After each round, assess your Distress Rating once more to see if it has come down, or if your feeling about the situation has changed *in any way*. There will usually be some shift, but if your rating has not changed at all, then repeat the sequence using the *following* sentence as you tap the Karate Chop Spot:

> *Even though I am stuck at (give rating number at which your Intensity Rating is stuck) I deeply and completely accept myself*

Your Reminder Phrase will be, "I am stuck at _____ ".

Doing this will usually bring your Distress Rating lower, when it does so, go back to your original sentence and continue with the next round.

A cardinal rule of this method is that you *must continue* the treatment until your Distress Rating has come down to a 2 or below, preferably to a zero. Some people settle for lowering it to say a 5 or a 4 and stop there because they are feeling better. This is not good enough. This method has a powerful carry-over effect into your actual life situation, but only if you work to get your rating *way down* to 2 or below. Anything less then that, while helpful, doesn't do the *major* job that is called for.

An important point:

As your Distress Rating lowers, change your sentence accordingly. For example, if you were sad and now feel less sad but still somewhat sad, now say something like:

"Even though I still feel *somewhat* sad, I deeply and completely accept myself", and use the abbreviated sentence "I feel somewhat sad (or a "little sad")" as you tap each spot. This way the sentence is kept *appropriate* to your changing feelings.

Once your Distress Rating has gone down to a *"2" or below* on all feelings involved in the situation, and if necessary on all aspects of this problem. If you are not readily reducing its intensity it is usually because you need to address another *aspect* of the problem in addition to the one you started with, and if you do you can then expect considerable carry-over into the actual situation. (For an excellent discussion of "aspects" see Gary Craig's EFT Manuals downloadable free from his website, www.emofree.com.). EFT is not simply a technique for "feeling better," it actually changes your *processing* of the situation, and its effect remains. Ordinarily there is an 80% carry-over into the actual situation, if not, then further work with EFT under the guidance of a trained professional, will usually handle the situation satisfactorily.

How To Use EFT To Prepare
For An *Anticipated* Situation Of Concern

(1) When you identify your concern (know that you are worried) bring your feelings of anger, fear, sadness (or any other emotions that apply) down to a "2" or below by using the method described above.

(2) Later the same day, check your Distress Rating once more (this is like taking your temperature), and if it is above a "2" (perhaps because of some input from the environment) immediately bring it down again to a "2" or below.

(3) Each morning before the upcoming event, as soon as you wake up check your Distress Rating again. If it is above a "2", bring it down to a "2" or below.

(4) Shortly before the anticipated situation takes place, check your Distress Rating again. If it is above a "2", bring it down immediately.

This should result in allowing you to be highly effective when you confront the actual situation.

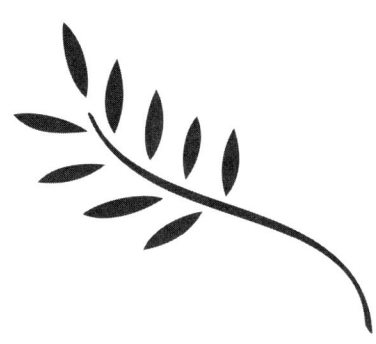